Virtual Clinical Excursions—Obstetrics-Pediatrics

for

Leifer:
Introduction to Maternity and Pediatric Nursing,
5th Edition

Virtual Clinical Excursions—Obstetrics-Pediatrics

for

Leifer:
Introduction to Maternity and Pediatric Nursing, 5th Edition

prepared by

Kelly Ann Crum, RN, MSN
Instructional Specialist
Lead Faculty
Curriculum Development/Maternal Child Nursing Specialty
Health Sciences and Nursing Department
University of Phoenix, Online
Phoenix, Arizona

Betty W. Hamlisch, RN, MS Health Education
Professor of Nursing
Tompkins Cortland Community College
Dryden, New York

software developed by

Wolfsong Informatics, LLC
Tucson, Arizona

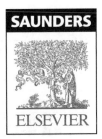

SAUNDERS

ELSEVIER

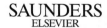

SAUNDERS
ELSEVIER

11830 Westline Industrial Dr.
St. Louis, Missouri 63146

VIRTUAL CLINICAL EXCURSIONS—OBSTETRICS-PEDIATRICS FOR
LEIFER: INTRODUCTION TO MATERNITY AND PEDIATRIC NURSING,
FIFTH EDITION

ISBN-13: 978-1-4160-4101-6
ISBN-10: 1-4160-4101-X

Copyright © 2007 by Saunders, an imprint of Elsevier Inc.

Notice

Knowledge and best practice in this field are constantly changing. As new research and experience broaden our knowledge, changes in practice, treatment and drug therapy may become necessary or appropriate. Readers are advised to check the most current information provided (i) on procedures featured or (ii) by the manufacturer of each product to be administered, to verify the recommended dose or formula, the method and duration of administration, and contraindications. It is the responsibility of the practitioner, relying on their own experience and knowledge of the patient, to make diagnoses, to determine dosages and the best treatment for each individual patient, and to take all appropriate safety precautions. To the fullest extent of the law, neither the Publisher nor the Authors assumes any liability for any injury and/or damage to persons or property arising out or related to any use of the material contained in this book.

ISBN-13: 978-1-4160-4101-6
ISBN-10: 1-4160-4101-X

Executive Editor: *Tom Wilhelm*
Managing Editor: *Jeff Downing*
Associate Developmental Editor: *Tiffany Trautwein*
Book Production Manager: *Gayle May*
Project Manager: *Tracey Schriefer*

Printed in the United States of America

Last digit is the print number: 9 8 7 6 5 4

*Workbook
prepared by*

Kelly Ann Crum, RN, MSN
Instructional Specialist
Lead Faculty
Curriculum Development/Maternal Child Nursing Specialty
Health Sciences and Nursing Department
University of Phoenix, Online
Phoenix, Arizona

Betty W. Hamlisch, RN, MS Health Education
Professor of Nursing
Tompkins Cortland Community College
Dryden, New York

Textbook

Gloria Leifer, MA, RN
Associate Professor, Obstetrics, Pediatrics, and Trauma Nursing
Riverside Community College
Riverside, California

Contents

Table of Contents
Leifer: Introduction to Maternity and Pediatric Nursing, 5th Edition

EFM - external fetal monitor

Unit V—The Child Needing Nursing Care

Unit VI—The Changing Health Care Environment

Appendixes

Getting Started

GETTING SET UP

■ **MINIMUM SYSTEM REQUIREMENTS**

WINDOWS®

Windows Vista™, XP, 2000 (Recommend Windows XP/2000)
Pentium® III processor (or equivalent) @ 600 MHz (Recommend 800 MHz or better)
256 MB of RAM (Recommend 1 GB or more for Windows Vista)
800 x 600 screen size (Recommend 1024 x 768)
Thousands of colors
12x CD-ROM drive
Soundblaster 16 soundcard compatibility
Stereo speakers or headphones

Note: Windows Vista and XP require administrator privileges for installation.

MACINTOSH®

MAC OS X (10.2 or higher)
Apple Power PC G3 @ 500 MHz or better
128 MB of RAM (Recommend 256 MB or more)
800 x 600 screen size (Recommend 1024 x 768)
Thousands of colors
12x CD-ROM drive
Stereo speakers or headphones

1

■ INSTALLATION INSTRUCTIONS

WINDOWS

1. Insert the *Virtual Clinical Excursions—Obstetrics-Pediatrics* CD-ROM.
2. The setup screen should appear automatically if the current product is not already installed. Windows Vista users may be asked to authorize additional security prompts.
3. Follow the onscreen instructions during the setup process.

    If the setup screen does *not* appear automatically (and *Virtual Clinical Excursions—Obstetrics-Pediatrics* has not been installed already):
    a. Click the **My Computer** icon on your desktop or on your Start menu.
    b. Double-click on your CD-ROM drive.
    c. If installation does not start at this point:
       (1) Click the **Start** icon on the taskbar and select the **Run** option.
       (2) Type d:\setup.exe (where "d:\" is your CD-ROM drive) and press **OK**.
       (3) Follow the onscreen instructions for installation.

MACINTOSH

1. Insert the *Virtual Clinical Excursions—Obstetrics-Pediatrics* CD in the CD-ROM drive. The disk icon will appear on your desktop.

2. Double-click on the disk icon.

3. Double-click on the VCEOBPE_MAC run file.

Note: Virtual Clinical Excursions—Obstetrics-Pediatrics for Macintosh does not have an installation setup and can only be run directly from the CD.

■ HOW TO USE VIRTUAL CLINICAL EXCURSIONS—OBSTETRICS-PEDIATRICS

WINDOWS

1. Double-click on the *Virtual Clinical Excursions—Obstetrics-Pediatrics* icon located on your desktop.
2. Or navigate to the program via the Windows Start menu.

Note: If your computer uses Windows Vista, right-click on the desktop shortcut and choose **Properties**. In the Compatability Mode, check the box for "Run as Administrator." Below is a screen capture to show what this looks like.

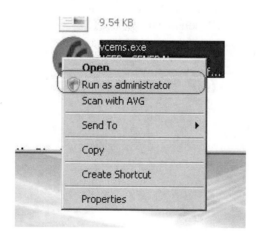

MACINTOSH

1. Insert the *Virtual Clinical Excursions—Obstetrics-Pediatrics* CD in the CD-ROM drive. The disk icon will appear on your desktop.

2. Double-click on the disk icon.

3. Double-click on the VCEOBPE_MAC run file.

■ SCREEN SETTINGS

For best results, your computer monitor resolution should be set at a minimum of 800 x 600. The number of colors displayed should be set to "thousands or higher" (High Color or 16 bit) or "millions of colors" (True Color or 24 bit).

Windows

1. From the **Start** menu, select **Control Panel** (on some systems, you will first go to **Settings**, then to **Control Panel**).
2. Double-click on the **Display** icon.
3. Click on the **Settings** tab.
4. Under **Screen resolution** use the slider bar to select **800 by 600 pixels**.
5. Access the **Colors** drop-down menu by clicking on the down arrow.
6. Select **High Color (16 bit)** or **True Color (24 bit)**.
7. Click on **OK**.
8. You may be asked to verify the setting changes. Click **Yes**.
9. You may be asked to restart your computer to accept the changes. Click **Yes**.

Macintosh

1. Select the **Monitors** control panel.
2. Select **800 x 600** (or similar) from the **Resolution** area.
3. Select **Thousands** or **Millions** from the **Color Depth** area.

■ WEB BROWSERS

Supported web browsers include Microsoft Internet Explorer (IE) version 6.0 or higher and Mozilla Firefox version 2.0 or higher. The supported browser for Macs running OS X is Mozilla Firefox.

If you use America Online® (AOL) for web access, you will need AOL version 4.0 or higher and one of the browsers listed above. Do not use earlier versions of AOL with earlier versions of IE, because you will have difficulty accessing many features.

For best results with AOL:
- Connect to the Internet using AOL version 4.0 or higher.
- Open a private chat within AOL (this allows the AOL client to remain open, without asking whether you wish to disconnect while minimized).
- Minimize AOL.
- Launch a recommended browser.

■ **TECHNICAL SUPPORT**

Technical support for this product is available between 7:30 a.m. and 7 p.m. (CST), Monday through Friday. Before calling, be sure that your computer meets the minimum system requirements to run this software. Inside the United States and Canada, call 1-800-692-9010. Outside North America, call 314-872-8370. You may also fax your questions to 314-523-4932 or contact Technical Support through e-mail: technical.support@elsevier.com.

Trademarks: Windows, Macintosh, Pentium, and America Online are registered trademarks.

Copyright © 2007 by Saunders, an imprint of Elsevier Inc.

All rights reserved. No part of this product may be reproduced or transmitted in any form or by any means, electronic or mechanical, including input or storage in any information system, without written permission from the publisher.

ACCESSING *Virtual Clinical Excursions—Obstetrics-Pediatrics* FROM EVOLVE

The product you have purchased is part of the Evolve family of online courses and learning resources. Please read the following information thoroughly to get started.

To access your instructor's course on Evolve:

Your instructor will provide you with the username and password needed to access this specific course on the Evolve Learning System. Once you have received this information, please follow these instructions:

1. Go to the Evolve student page (http://evolve.elsevier.com/student).

2. Enter your username and password in the **Login to My Evolve** area and click the **Login** button.

3. You will be taken to your personalized **My Evolve** page, where the course will be listed in the **My Courses** module.

TECHNICAL REQUIREMENTS

To use an Evolve course, you will need access to a computer that is connected to the Internet and equipped with web browser software that supports frames. For optimal performance, it is recommended that you have speakers and use a high-speed Internet connection. However, slower dial-up modems (56 K minimum) are acceptable.

Whichever browser you use, the browser preferences must be set to enable cookies and the cache must be set to reload every time.

Enable Cookies

Browser	Steps
Internet Explorer (IE) 6.0 or higher	1. Select **Tools → Internet Options**. 2. Select **Privacy** tab. 3. Use the slider (slide down) to **Accept All Cookies**. 4. Click **OK**. -OR- 3. Click the **Advanced** button. 4. Click the check box next to **Override Automatic Cookie Handling**. 5. Click the **Accept** radio buttons under **First-party Cookies** and **Third-party Cookies**. 6. Click **OK**.
Mozilla Firefox 2.0 or higher	1. Select **Tools → Options**. 2. Select the **Privacy** icon. 3. Click to expand Cookies. 4. Select **Allow sites to set cookies**. 5. Click **OK**.

Set Cache to Always Reload a Page

Browser	Steps
Internet Explorer (IE) 6.0 or higher	1. Select **Tools → Internet Options**. 2. Select **General** tab. 3. Go to the **Temporary Internet Files** and click the **Settings** button. 4. Select the radio button for **Every visit to the page** and click **OK** when complete.
Mozilla Firefox 2.0 or higher	1. Select **Tools → Options**. 2. Select the **Privacy** icon. 3. Click to expand Cache. 4. Set the value to "**0**" in the **Use up to: __ MB of disk space for the cache** field. 5. Click **OK**.

Plug-Ins

 Adobe Acrobat Reader—With the free Acrobat Reader software, you can view and print Adobe PDF files. Many Evolve products offer student and instructor manuals, checklists, and more in this format!

Download at: http://www.adobe.com

 Apple QuickTime—Install this to hear word pronunciations, heart and lung sounds, and many other helpful audio clips within Evolve Online Courses!

Download at: http://www.apple.com

 Adobe Flash Player—This player will enhance your viewing of many Evolve web pages, as well as educational short-form to long-form animation within the Evolve Learning System!

Download at: http://www.adobe.com

 Adobe Shockwave Player—Shockwave is best for viewing the many interactive learning activities within Evolve Online Courses!

Download at: http://www.adobe.com

 Microsoft Word Viewer—With this viewer, Microsoft Word users can share documents with those who don't have Word, and users without Word can open and view Word documents. Many Evolve products have testbank, student and instructor manuals, and other documents available for downloading and viewing on your own computer!

Download at: http://www.microsoft.com

 Microsoft PowerPoint Viewer—With this viewer, you can access PowerPoint 97, 2000, and 2002 presentations even if you don't have PowerPoint. Many Evolve products have slides available for downloading and viewing on your own computer!

Download at: http://www.microsoft.com

SUPPORT INFORMATION

Live phone support is available to customers in the United States and Canada at **800-401-9962** from 7:30 a.m. to 7 p.m. (CST), Monday through Friday. Support is also available through email at evolve-support@elsevier.com.

Online 24/7 support can be accessed on the Evolve website (http://evolve.elsevier.com). Resources include:

- Guided tours
- Tutorials
- Frequently asked questions (FAQs)
- Online copies of course user guides
- And much more!

A QUICK TOUR

Welcome to *Virtual Clinical Excursions—Obstetrics-Pediatrics*, a virtual hospital setting in which you can work with multiple complex patient simulations and also learn to access and evaluate the information resources that are essential for high-quality patient care. The virtual hospital, Pacific View Regional Hospital, has realistic architecture and access to patient rooms, a Nurses' Station, and a Medication Room.

■ BEFORE YOU START

Make sure you have your textbook nearby when you use the *Virtual Clinical Excursions— Obstetrics-Pediatrics* CD. You will want to consult topic areas in your textbook frequently while working with the CD and using this workbook.

■ HOW TO SIGN IN

- Enter your name on the Student Nurse identification badge.
- Next, click the down arrow next to **Select Floor**. For this quick tour, choose **Obstetrics**.
- Now click the down arrow next to **Select Period of Care**. This drop-down menu gives you four periods of care from which to choose. In Periods of Care 1 through 3, you can actively engage in patient assessment, entry of data in the electronic patient record (EPR), and medication administration. Period of Care 4 presents the day in review. Highlight and click the appropriate period of care. (For this quick tour, choose **Period of Care 1: 0730-0815**.)
- Click **Go**. This takes you to the Patient List screen (see example on page 11). Note that the virtual time is provided in the box at the lower left corner of the screen (0730, since we chose Period of Care 1).

Note: If you choose to work during Period of Care 4: 1900-2000, the Patient List screen is skipped since you are not able to visit patients or administer medications during the shift. Instead, you are taken directly to the Nurses' Station, where the records of all the patients on the floor are available for your review.

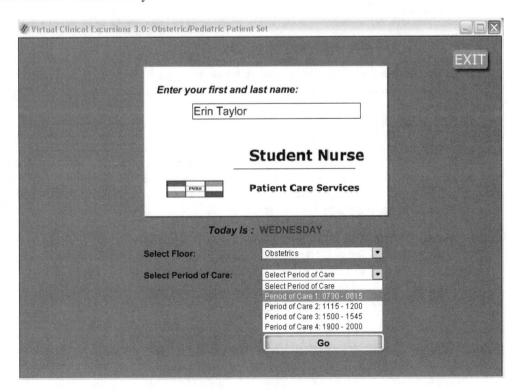

■ PATIENT LIST

OBSTETRICS UNIT

Dorothy Grant (Room 201)
30-week intrauterine pregnancy—A 25-year-old Caucasian multipara admitted with abdominal trauma following a domestic violence incident. Her complications include preterm labor and extensive social issues such as acquiring safe housing for her family upon discharge.

Stacey Crider (Room 202)
27-week intrauterine pregnancy—A 21-year-old Native American primigravida admitted for intravenous tocolysis, bacterial vaginosis, and poorly controlled insulin-dependent gestational diabetes. Strained family relationships and social isolation complicate this patient's ability to comply with strict dietary requirements and prenatal care.

Kelly Brady (Room 203)
26-week intrauterine pregnancy—A 35-year-old Caucasian primigravida urgently admitted for progressive symptoms of preeclampsia. A history of inadequate coping with major life stressors leave her at risk for a recurrence of depression as she faces a diagnosis of HELLP syndrome and the delivery of a severely premature infant.

Maggie Gardner (Room 204)
22-week intrauterine pregnancy—A 41-year-old African-American multigravida admitted for a high-risk pregnancy evaluation and rule out diagnosis of systemic lupus erythematosus. Coping with chronic pain, fatigue, and a history of multiple miscarriages contribute to an anxiety disorder and the need for social service intervention.

Gabriela Valenzuela (Room 205)
34-week intrauterine pregnancy—A 21-year-old Hispanic primigravida with a history of mitral valve prolapse admitted for uterine cramping and vaginal bleeding suggestive of placental abruption following an unrestrained motor vehicle accident. Her needs include staff support for an unprepared-for labor and possible preterm birth.

Laura Wilson (Room 206)
37-week intrauterine pregnancy—An 18-year-old Caucasian primigravida urgently admitted after being found unconscious at home. Her complications include HIV-positive status and chronic polysubstance abuse. Unrealistic expectations of parenthood and living with a chronic illness combined with strained family relations prompt comprehensive social and psychiatric evaluations initiated on the day of simulation.

PEDIATRICS UNIT

George Gonzalez (Room 301)
Diabetic ketoacidosis—An 11-year-old Hispanic male admitted for stabilization of blood glucose level and diabetic re-education associated with his diagnosis of type 1 diabetes mellitus. This patient's poor compliance with insulin therapy and dietary regime have resulted in frequent and repeated hospital admissions for DKA.

Tommy Douglas (Room 302)
Traumatic brain injury—A 6-year-old Caucasian male transferred from the Pediatric Intensive Care Unit in preparation for organ donation. This patient is status post ventriculostomy with negative intracerebral blood flow and requires extensive hemodynamic monitoring and support, along with compassionate family care.

Carrie Richards (Room 303)
Bronchiolitis—A 3½-month-old African-American female admitted with respiratory distress due to respiratory syncytial virus, along with dehydration and an inadequate nutritional status. Parent education and support are among her primary needs.

Stephanie Brown (Room 304)
Meningitis—A 3-year-old African-American female with a history of spastic cerebral palsy
admitted for intravenous antibiotic therapy, neurologic monitoring, and support for a diagnosis
of acute meningitis. Maintenance of physical and occupational programs addressing her mobil-
ity limitations complicate her acute care stay.

Tiffany Sheldon (Room 305)
Anorexia nervosa—A 14-year-old Caucasian female admitted for dehydration, electrolyte
imbalance, and malnutrition following a syncope episode at home. This patient has a history of
eating disorders, which have resulted in multiple hospital admissions and strained family
dynamics between mother and daughter.

■ HOW TO SELECT A PATIENT

- You can choose one or more patients to work with from the Patient List by checking the box
  to the left of the patient name(s). For this quick tour, select Dorothy Grant. (In order to
  receive a scorecard for a patient, the patient must be selected before proceeding to the
  Nurses' Station.)
- Click on **Get Report** to the right of the medical records number (MRN) to view a summary
  of the patient's care during the 12-hour period before your arrival on the unit.
- After reviewing the report, click on **Go to Nurses' Station** in the right lower corner to begin
  your care. (*Note:* If you have been assigned to care for multiple patients, you can click on
  Return to Patient List to select and review the report for each additional patient before
  going to the Nurses' Station.)

Note: Even though the Patient List is initially skipped when you sign in to work for Period of
Care 4, you can still access this screen if you wish to review the shift report for any of the
patients. To do so, simply click on **Patient List** near the top left corner of the Nurses' Station (or
click on the clipboard to the left of the Kardex). Then click on **Get Report** for the patient(s)
whose care you are reviewing. This may be done during any period of care.

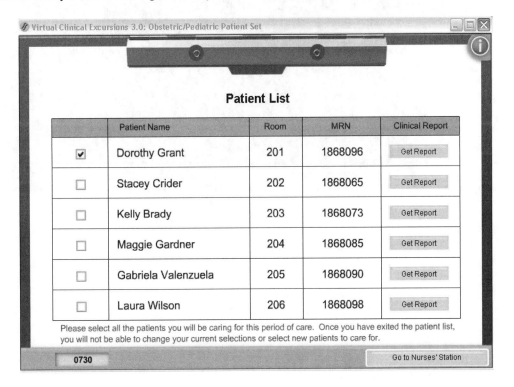

■ HOW TO FIND A PATIENT'S RECORDS

NURSES' STATION

Within the Nurses' Station, you will see:

1. A clipboard that contains the patient list for that floor.
2. A chart rack with patient charts labeled by room number, a notebook labeled Kardex, and a notebook labeled MAR (Medication Administration Record).
3. A desktop computer with access to the Electronic Patient Record (EPR).
4. A tool bar across the top of the screen that can also be used to access the Patient List, EPR, Chart, MAR, and Kardex. This tool bar is also accessible from each patient's room.
5. A Drug Guide containing information about the medications you are able to administer to your patients.
6. A tool bar across the bottom of the screen that can be used to access the Floor Map, patient rooms, Medication Room, and Drug Guide.

As you run your cursor over an item, it will be highlighted. To select, simply double-click on the item. As you use these resources, you will always be able to return to the Nurses' Station by clicking on the **Return to Nurses' Station** bar located in the right lower corner of your screen.

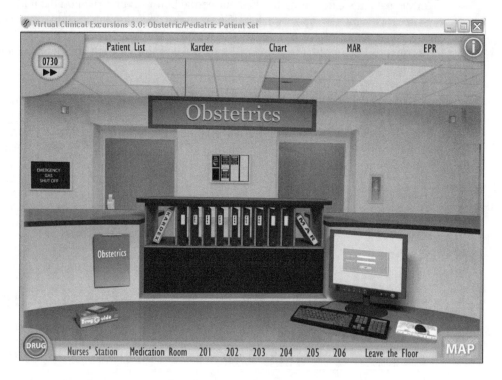

MEDICATION ADMINISTRATION RECORD (MAR)

The MAR icon located on the tool bar at the top of your screen accesses current 24-hour medications for each patient. Click on the icon and the MAR will open. (*Note:* You can also access the MAR by clicking on the MAR notebook on the far right side of the book rack in the center of the screen.) Within the MAR, tabs on the right side of the screen allow you to select patients by room number. Be careful to make sure you select the correct tab number for *your* patient rather than simply reading the first record that appears after the MAR opens. Each MAR sheet lists the following:

- Medications
- Route and dosage of each medication
- Times of administration of each medication

Note: The MAR changes each day. Expired MARs are stored in the patients' charts.

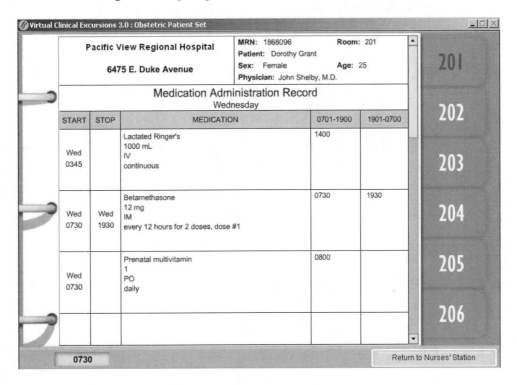

CHARTS

To access patient charts, either click on the **Chart** icon at the top of your screen or anywhere within the chart rack in the center of the Nurses' Station screen. When the close-up view appears, the individual charts are labeled by room number. To open a chart, click on the room number of the patient whose chart you wish to review. The patient's name and allergies will appear on the left side of the screen, along with a list of tabs on the right side of the screen, allowing you to view the following data:

- Allergies
- Physician's Orders
- Physician's Notes
- Nurse's Notes
- Laboratory Reports
- Diagnostic Reports
- Surgical Reports
- Consultations

- Patient Education
- History and Physical
- Nursing Admission
- Expired MARs
- Consents
- Mental Health
- Admissions
- Emergency Department

Information appears in real time. The entries are in reverse chronologic order, so use the down arrow at the right side of each chart page to scroll down to view previous entries. Flip from tab to tab to view multiple data fields or click on **Return to Nurses' Station** in the lower right corner of the screen to exit the chart.

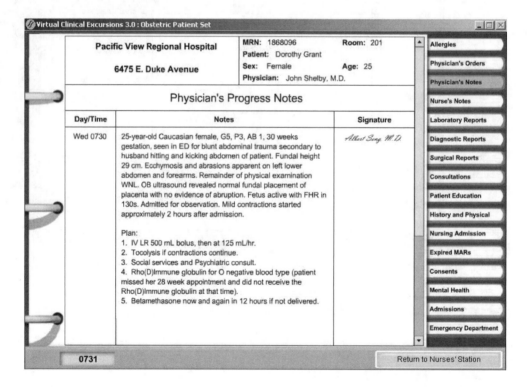

ELECTRONIC PATIENT RECORD (EPR)

The EPR can be accessed from the computer in the Nurses' Station or from the EPR icon located in the tool bar at the top of your screen. To access a patient's EPR:

- Click on either the computer screen or the **EPR** icon.
- Your username and password are automatically filled in.
- Click on **Login** to enter the EPR.
- *Note:* Like the MAR, the EPR is arranged numerically. Thus when you enter, you are initially shown the records of the patient in the lowest room number on the floor. To view the correct data for *your* patient, remember to select the correct room number, using the drop-down menu for the Patient field at the top left corner of the screen.

The EPR used in Pacific View Regional Hospital represents a composite of commercial versions being used in hospitals. You can access the EPR:

- to review existing data for a patient (by room number).
- to enter data you collect while working with a patient.

The EPR is updated daily, so no matter what day or part of a shift you are working, there will be a current EPR with the patient's data from the past days of the current hospital stay. This type of simulated EPR allows you to examine how data for different attributes have changed over time, as well as to examine data for all of a patient's attributes at a particular time. The EPR is fully functional (as it is in a real-life hospital). You can enter such data as blood pressure, breath sounds, and certain treatments. The EPR will not, however, allow you to enter data for a previous time period. Use the arrows at the bottom of the screen to move forward and backward in time.

Virtual Clinical Excursions 3.0 : Obstetric Patient Set					_ □ ×
Patient: 201 ▼ **Category:** Vital Signs ▼					**0731**
Name: Dorothy Grant	Wed 0345	Wed 0400	Wed 0500	Code Meanings	
PAIN: LOCATION	A	A	A	A	Abdomen
PAIN: RATING	1	1	2-3	Ar	Arm
PAIN: CHARACTERISTICS	A	D	I	B	Back
PAIN: VOCAL CUES		NN	NN	C	Chest
PAIN: FACIAL CUES			FC2	Ft	Foot
PAIN: BODILY CUES				H	Head
PAIN: SYSTEM CUES	NN			Hd	Hand
PAIN: FUNCTIONAL EFFECTS				L	Left
PAIN: PREDISPOSING FACTORS		NN	NN	Lg	Leg
PAIN: RELIEVING FACTORS		NN	NN	Lw	Lower
PCA				N	Neck
TEMPERATURE (F)		97.6		NN	See Nurses notes
TEMPERATURE (C)				OS	Operative site
MODE OF MEASUREMENT		O		Or	See Physicians orders
SYSTOLIC PRESSURE		126		PN	See Progress notes
DIASTOLIC PRESSURE		66		R	Right
BP MODE OF MEASUREMENT		NIBP		Up	Upper
HEART RATE		72			
RESPIRATORY RATE		18			
SpO2 (%)					
BLOOD GLUCOSE					
WEIGHT					
HEIGHT					
	◄		►	Exit EPR	

At the top of the EPR screen, you can choose patients by their room numbers. In addition, you have access to 17 different categories of patient data. To change patients or data categories, click the down arrow to the right of the room number or category.

The categories of patient data in the EPR as as follows:

- Vital Signs
- Respiratory
- Cardiovascular
- Neurologic
- Gastrointestinal
- Excretory
- Musculoskeletal
- Integumentary
- Reproductive
- Psychosocial
- Wounds and Drains
- Activity
- Hygiene and Comfort
- Safety
- Nutrition
- IV
- Intake and Output

Remember, each hospital selects its own codes. The codes used in the EPR at Pacific View Regional Hospital may be different from ones you have seen in your clinical rotations. Take some time to acquaint yourself with the codes. Within the Vital Signs category, click on any item in the left column (e.g., Pain: Characteristics). In the far-right column, you will see a list of code meanings for the possible findings and/or descriptors for that assessment area.

You will use the codes to record the data you collect as you work with patients. Click on the box in the last time column to the right of any item and wait for the code meanings applicable to that entry to appear. Select the appropriate code to describe your assessment findings and type it in the box. (*Note:* If no cursor appears within the box, click on the box again until the blue shading disappears and the blinking cursor appears.) Once the data are typed in this box, they are entered into the patient's record for this period of care only.

To leave the EPR, click on **Exit EPR** in the bottom right corner of the screen.

■ VISITING A PATIENT

From the Nurses' Station, click on the room number of the patient you wish to visit (in the tool bar at the bottom of your screen). Once you are inside the room, you will see a still photo of your patient in the top left corner. To verify that this is the correct patient, click on the **Check Armband** icon to the right of the photo. The patient's identification data will appear. If you click on **Check Allergies** (the next icon to the right), a list of the patient's allergies (if any) will replace the photo.

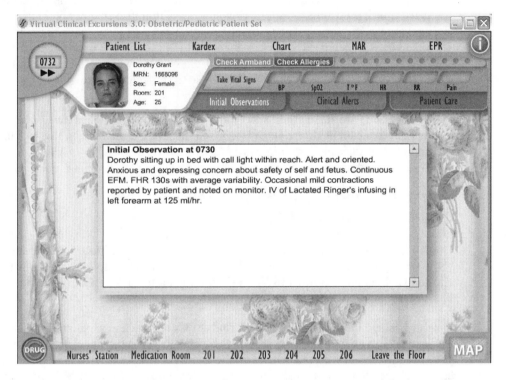

Also located in the patient's room are multiple icons you can use to assess the patient or the patient's medications. A virtual clock is provided in the upper left corner of the room to monitor your progress in real time. (*Note:* The fast-forward icon within the virtual clock will advance the time by 2-minute intervals when clicked.)

- The tool bar across the top of the screen allows you to check the **Patient List**, access the **EPR** to check or enter data, and view the patient's **Chart**, **MAR**, or **Kardex**.

- The **Take Vital Signs** icon allows you to measure the patient's up-to-the-minute blood pressure, oxygen saturation, temperature, heart rate, respiratory rate, and pain level.

- Each time you enter a patient's room, you are given an Initial Observation report to review (in the text box under the patient's photo). These notes are provided to give you a "look" at the patient as if you had just stepped into the room. You can also click on the **Initial Observations** icon to return to this box from other views within the patient's room. To the right of this icon is **Clinical Alerts**, a resource that allows you to make decisions about priority medication interventions based on emerging data collected in real time. Check this screen throughout your period of care to avoid missing critical information related to recently ordered or STAT medications.

- Clicking on **Patient Care** opens up three specific learning environments within the patient room: **Physical Assessment**, **Nurse-Client Interactions**, and **Medication Administration**.

- To perform a **Physical Assessment**, choose a body area (such as **Head & Neck**) from the column of yellow buttons. This activates a list of system subcategories for that body area (e.g., see **Sensory**, **Neurologic**, etc. in the green boxes). After you select the system you wish to evaluate, a brief description of the assessment findings will appear in a box to the right. A still photo provides a "snapshot" of how an assessment of this area might be done or what the finding might look like. For every body area, you can also click on **Equipment** on the right side of the screen.

- To the right of the Physical Assessment icon is **Nurse-Client Interactions**. Clicking on this icon will reveal the times and titles of any videos available for viewing. (*Note:* If the video you wish to see is not listed, this means you have not yet reached the correct virtual time to view that video. Check the virtual clock; you may return to access the video once its designated time has occurred—as long as you do so within the same period of care. Or you can click on the fast-forward icon within the virtual clock to advance the time by 2-minute intervals. You will then need to click again on **Patient Care** and **Nurse-Client Interactions** to refresh the screen.) To view a listed video, click on the white arrow to the right of the video title. Use the control buttons below the video to start, stop, pause, rewind, or fast-forward the action or to mute the sound.

- **Medication Administration** is the pathway that allows you to review and administer medications to a patient after you have prepared them in the Medication Room. This process is addressed further in *How to Prepare Medications* (pages 19-20), in *Medications* (pages 26-30) For additional hands-on practice, see *Reducing Medication Errors* (pages 37-41).

■ HOW TO QUIT, CHANGE PATIENTS, CHANGE FLOORS, OR CHANGE PERIODS OF CARE

How to Quit: From most screens, you may click the **Leave the Floor** icon on the bottom tool bar to the right of the patient room numbers. (*Note:* From some screens, you will first need to click an **Exit** button or **Return to Nurses' Station** before clicking **Leave the Floor**.) When the Floor Menu appears, click **Exit** to leave the program.

How to Change Patients, Floors, or Periods of Care: To change patients, simply click on the new patient's room number. (You cannot receive a scorecard for a new patient, however, unless you have already selected that patient on the Patient List screen.) To change to a new period of care, to change floors, or to restart the virtual clock, click on **Leave the Floor** and then on **Restart the Program**.

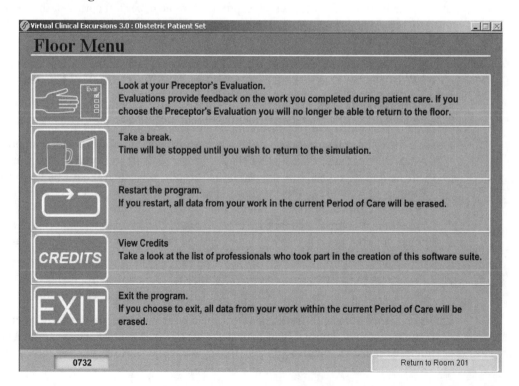

■ HOW TO PREPARE MEDICATIONS

From the Nurses' Station or the patient's room, you can access the Medication Room by clicking on the icon in the tool bar at the bottom of your screen to the left of the patient room numbers.

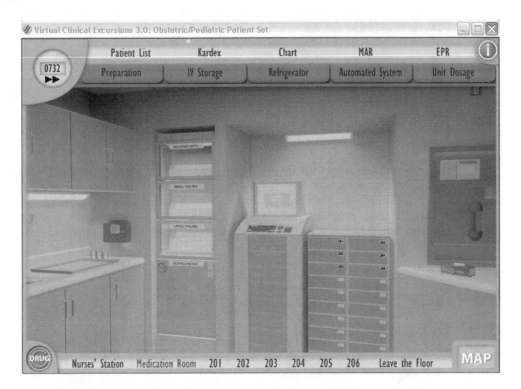

In the Medication Room you have access to the following (from left to right):

- A preparation area is located on the counter under the cabinets. To begin the medication preparation process, click on the tray on the counter or click on the **Preparation** icon at the top of the screen. The next screen leads you through a specific sequence (called the Preparation Wizard) to prepare medications one at a time for administration to a patient. However, no medication has been selected at this time. We will do this while working with a patient in *A Detailed Tour*. To exit this screen, click on **View Medication Room**.

- To the right of the cabinets (and above the refrigerator), IV storage bins are provided. Click on the bins themselves or on the **IV Storage** icon at the top of the screen. The bins are labeled **Microinfusion**, **Small Volume**, and **Large Volume**. Click on an individual bin to see a list of its contents. If you needed to prepare an IV medication at this time, you could click on the medication and its label would appear to the right under the patient's name. (*Note:* You can **Open** and **Close** any medication label by clicking the appropriate icon.) Next, you would click **Put Medication on Tray**. If you ever change your mind or decide that you have put the incorrect medication on the tray, you can reverse your actions by highlighting the medication on the tray and then clicking **Put Medication in Bin**. Click **Close Bin** in the right bottom corner to exit. **View Medication Room** brings you back to a full view of the entire room.

- A refrigerator is located under the IV storage bins to hold any medications that must be stored below room temperature. Click on the refrigerator door or on the **Refrigerator** icon at the top of the screen. Then click on the close-up view of the door to access the medications. When you are finished, click **Close Door** and then **View Medication Room**.

- To prepare controlled substances, click the **Automated System** icon at the top of the screen or click the computer monitor located to the right of the IV storage bins. A login screen will appear; your name and password are automatically filled in. Click **Login**. Select the patient for whom you wish to access medications; then select the correct medication drawer to open (they are stored alphabetically). Click **Open Drawer**, highlight the proper medication, and choose **Put Medication on Tray**. When you are finished, click **Close Drawer** and then **View Medication Room**.

- Next to the Automated System is a set of drawers identified by patient room number. To access these, click on the drawers or on the **Unit Dosage** icon at the top of the screen. This provides a close-up view of the drawers. To open a drawer, click on the room number of the patient you are working with. Next, click on the medication you would like to prepare for the patient, and a label will appear, listing the medication strength, units, and dosage per unit. To exit, click **Close Drawer**; then click **View Medication Room**.

At any time, you can learn about a medication you wish to prepare for a patient by clicking on the **Drug** icon in the bottom left corner of the medication room screen or by clicking the **Drug Guide** book on the counter to the right of the unit dosage drawers. The **Drug Guide** provides information about the medications commonly included in nursing drug handbooks. Nutritional supplements and maintenance intravenous fluid preparations are not included. Highlight a medication in the alphabetical list; relevant information about the drug will appear in the screen below. To exit, click **Return to Medication Room**.

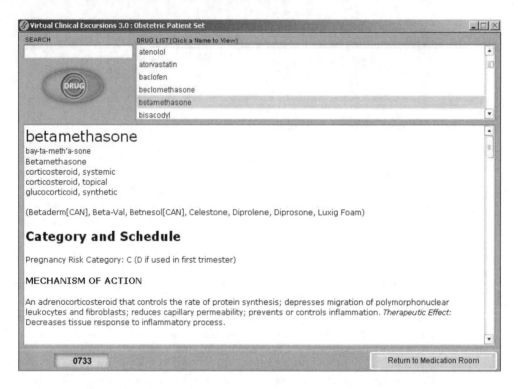

To access the MAR to review the medications ordered for a patient, click on the **MAR** icon located in the tool bar at the top of your screen and then click on the correct tab for your patient's room number. You may also click the **Review MAR** icon in the tool bar at the bottom of your screen from inside each medication storage area.

After you have chosen and prepared medications, go to the patient's room to administer them by clicking on the room number in the bottom tool bar. Inside the patient's room, click **Patient Care** and then **Medication Administration** and follow the proper administration sequence.

■ **PRECEPTOR'S EVALUATIONS**

When you have finished a session, click on **Leave the Floor** to go to the Floor Menu. At this point, you can click on the top icon (**Look at Your Preceptor's Evaluation**) to receive a score-card that provides feedback on the work you completed during patient care.

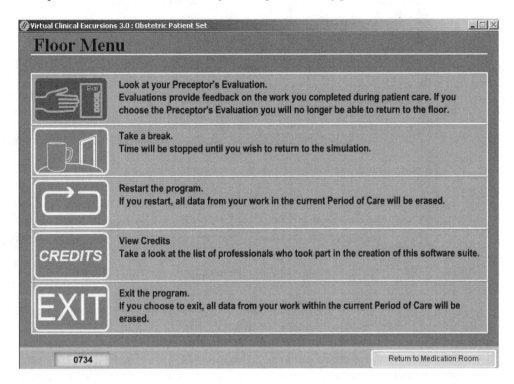

Evaluations are available for each patient you selected when you signed in for the current period of care. Click on the **Medication Scorecard** icon to see an example.

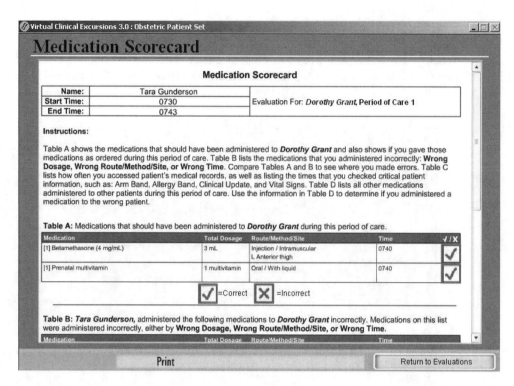

The scorecard compares the medications you administered to a patient during a period of care with what should have been administered. Table A lists the correct medications. Table B lists any medications that were administered incorrectly.

Remember, not every medication listed on the MAR should necessarily be given. For example, a patient might have an allergy to a drug that was ordered, or a medication might have been improperly transcribed to the MAR. Predetermined medication "errors" embedded within the program challenge you to exercise critical thinking skills and professional judgment when deciding to administer a medication, just as you would in a real hospital. Use all your available resources, such as the patient's chart and the MAR, to make your decision.

Table C lists the resources that were available to assist you in medication administration. It also documents whether and when you accessed these resources. For example, did you check the patient armband or perform a check of vital signs? If so, when?

You can click **Print** to get a copy of this report if needed. When you have finished reviewing the scorecard, click **Return to Evaluations** and then **Return to Menu**.

■ FLOOR MAP

To get a general sense of your location within the hospital, you can click on the **Map** icon found in the lower right corner of most of the screens in the *Virtual Clinical Excursions—Obstetrics-Pediatrics* program. (*Note:* If you are following this quick tour step by step, you will need to **Restart the Program** from the Floor Menu, sign in again, and go to the Nurses' Station to access the map.) When you click the **Map** icon, a floor map appears, showing the layout of the floor you are currently on, as well as a directory of the patients and services on that floor. As you move your cursor over the directory list, the location of each room is highlighted on the map (and vice versa). The floor map can be accessed from the Nurses' Station, Medication Room, and each patient's room.

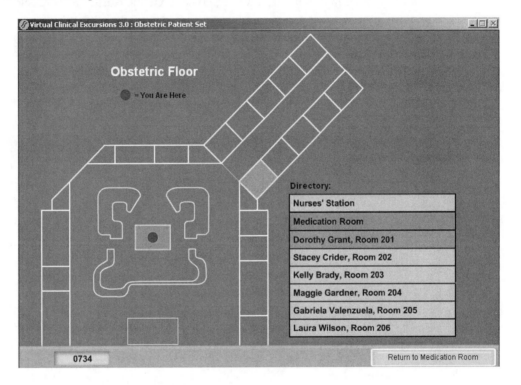

A DETAILED TOUR

If you wish to more thoroughly understand the capabilities of *Virtual Clinical Excursions—Obstetrics-Pediatrics*, take a detailed tour by completing the following section. During this tour, we will work with a specific patient to introduce you to all the different components and learning opportunities available within the software.

■ WORKING WITH A PATIENT

Sign in to work on the Obstetrics Floor for Period of Care 1 (0730-0815). From the Patient List, select Dorothy Grant in Room 201; however, do not go to the Nurses' Station yet.

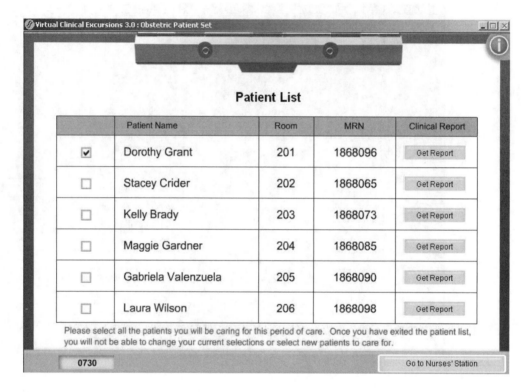

Patient Name	Room	MRN	Clinical Report
☑ Dorothy Grant	201	1868096	Get Report
☐ Stacey Crider	202	1868065	Get Report
☐ Kelly Brady	203	1868073	Get Report
☐ Maggie Gardner	204	1868085	Get Report
☐ Gabriela Valenzuela	205	1868090	Get Report
☐ Laura Wilson	206	1868098	Get Report

Please select all the patients you will be caring for this period of care. Once you have exited the patient list, you will not be able to change your current selections or select new patients to care for.

0730   Go to Nurses' Station

■ REPORT

In hospitals, when one shift ends and another begins, the outgoing nurse who attended a patient will give a verbal and sometimes a written summary of that patient's condition to the incoming nurse who will assume care for the patient. This summary is called a report and is an important source of data to provide an overview of a patient. Your first task is to get the clinical report on Dorothy Grant. To do this, click **Get Report** in the far right column in this patient's row. From a brief review of this summary, identify the problems and areas of concern that you will need to address for this patient.

When you have finished noting any areas of concern, click **Go to Nurses' Station**.

■ CHARTS

You can access Dorothy Grant's chart from the Nurses' Station or from the patient's room (201).
From the Nurses' Station, click on the chart rack or on the **Chart** icon in the tool bar at the top
of your screen. Next, click on the chart labeled **201** to open the medical record for Dorothy
Grant. Click on the **Emergency Department** tab to view a record of why this patient was
admitted.

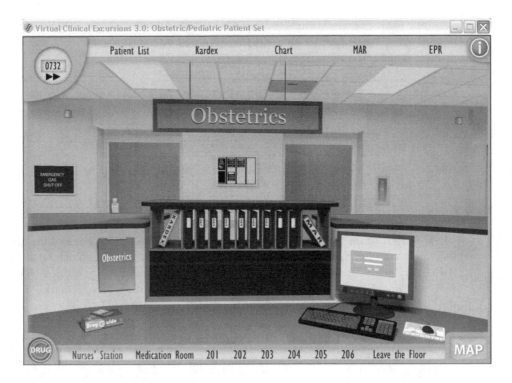

How many days has Dorothy Grant been in the hospital?

What tests were done upon her arrival in the Emergency Department and why?

What was the reason for her admission?

You should also click on **Surgical Reports** to learn whether any procedures were performed and
when. Finally, review the **Nursing Admission** and **History and Physical** to learn about the
health history of this patient. When you are done reviewing the chart, click **Return to Nurses'
Station**.

■ MEDICATIONS

Open the Medication Administration Record (MAR) by clicking on the **MAR** icon in the tool bar at the top of your screen. *Remember:* The MAR automatically opens to the first occupied room number on the floor—which is not necessarily your patient's room number! Since you need to access Dorothy Grant's MAR, click on tab **201** (her room number). Always make sure you are giving the *Right Drug to the Right Patient!*

Examine the list of medications ordered for Dorothy Grant. In the table below, list the medications that need to be given during this period of care (0730-0815). For each medication, note the dosage, route, and time to be given.

Time	Medication	Dosage	Route

Click on **Return to Nurses' Station**. Next, click on **201** on the bottom tool bar and then verify that you are indeed in Dorothy Grant's room. Select **Clinical Alerts** (the icon to the right of Initial Observations) to check for any emerging data that might affect your medication administration priorities. Next, go to the patient's chart (click on the **Chart** icon; then click on **201**). When the chart opens, select the **Physician's Orders** tab.

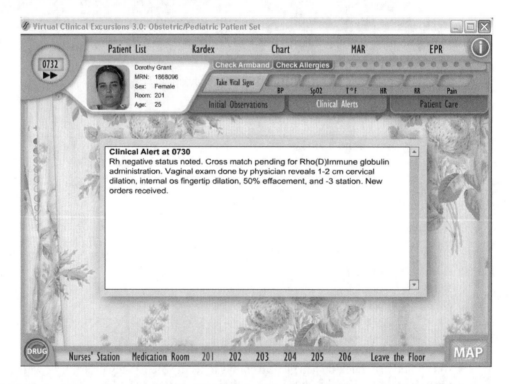

Review the orders. Have any new medications been ordered? Return to the MAR (click **Return to Room 201**; then click **MAR**). Verify that the new medications have been correctly transcribed to the MAR. Mistakes are sometimes made in the transcription process in the hospital setting, and it is sound practice to double-check any new order.

Are there any patient assessments you will need to perform before administering these medications? If so, return to Room 201 and click on **Patient Care** and then **Physical Assessment** to complete those assessments before proceeding.

Now click on the **Medication Room** icon in the tool bar at the bottom of your screen to locate and prepare the medications for Dorothy Grant.

In the Medication Room, you must access the medications for Dorothy Grant from the specific dispensing system in which each medication is stored. Locate each medication that needs to be given in this time period and click on **Put Medication on Tray** as appropriate. (*Hint:* Look in **Unit Dosage** drawer first.) When you are finished, click on **Close Drawer** and then on **View Medication Room**. Now click on the medication tray on the counter on the left side of the medication room screen to begin preparing the medications you have selected. (*Remember:* You can also click **Preparation** in the tool bar at the top of screen.)

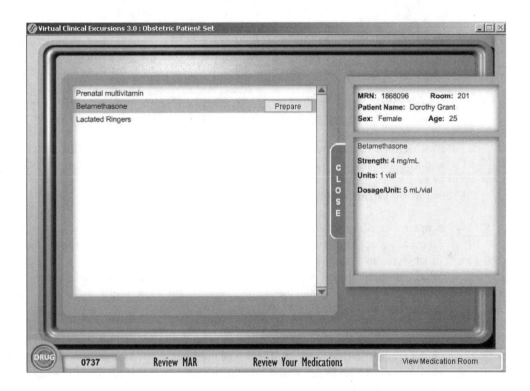

In the preparation area, you should see a list of the medications you put on the tray in the previous steps. Click on the first medication and then click **Prepare**. Follow the onscreen instructions of the Preparation Wizard, providing any data requested. As an example, let's follow the preparation process for betamethasone, one of the medications due to be administered to Dorothy Grant during this period of care. To begin, click on **Betamethasone**; then click **Prepare**. Now work through the Preparation Wizard sequence as detailed below:

> Amount of medication in the ampule: 5 mL.
> Enter the amount of medication you will draw up into a syringe: **3** mL.
> Click **Next**.
> Select the patient you wish to set aside the medication for: **Room 201, Dorothy Grant**.
> Click **Finish**.
> Click **Return to Medication Room**.

Follow this same basic process for the other medications due to be administered to Dorothy Grant during this period of care. (*Hint:* Look in **IV Storage** and **Automated System**.)

PREPARATION WIZARD EXCEPTIONS

- Some medications in *Virtual Clinical Excursions—Obstetrics-Pediatrics* are prepared by the pharmacy (e.g., IV antibiotics) and taken to the patient room as a whole. This is common practice in most hospitals.
- Blood products are not administered by students through the *Virtual Clinical Excursions—Obstetrics-Pediatrics* simulations since blood administration follows specific protocols not covered in this program.
- The *Virtual Clinical Excursions—Obstetrics-Pediatrics* simulations do not allow for mixing more than one type of medication, such as regular and Lente insulins, in the same syringe. In the clinical setting, when multiple types of insulin are ordered for a patient, the regular insulin is drawn up first, followed by the longer-acting insulin. Insulin is always administered in a special unit-marked syringe.

Now return to Room 201 (click on **201** on the bottom tool bar) to administer Dorothy Grant's medications.

At any time during the medication administration process, you can perform a further review of systems, take vital signs, check information contained within the chart, or verify patient identity and allergies. Inside Dorothy Grant's room, click **Take Vital Signs**. (*Note:* These findings change over time to reflect the temporal changes you would find in a patient similar to Dorothy Grant.)

When you have gathered all the data you need, click on **Patient Care** and then select **Medication Administration**. Any medications you prepared in the previous steps should be listed on the left side of your screen. Let's continue the administration process with the betamethasone ordered for Dorothy Grant. Click to highlight **Betamethasone** in the list of medications. Next, click on the down arrow to the right of **Select** and choose **Administer** from the drop-down menu. This will activate the Administration Wizard. Complete the Wizard sequence as follows:

- Route: **Injection**
- Method: **Intramuscular**
- Site: **Any**
- Click **Administer to Patient** arrow.
- Would you like to document this administration in the MAR? **Yes**
- Click **Finish** arrow.

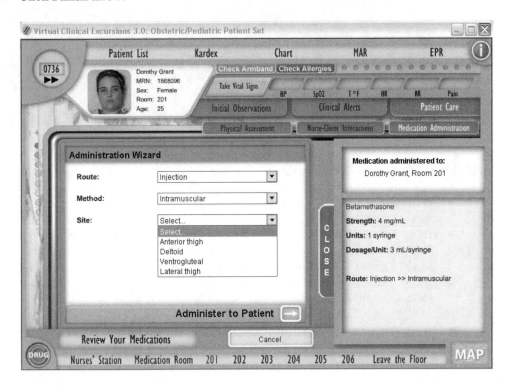

Your selections are recorded by a tracking system and evaluated on a Medication Scorecard stored under Preceptor's Evaluations. This scorecard can be viewed, printed, and given to your instructor. To access the Preceptor's Evaluations, click on **Leave the Floor**. When the Floor Menu appears, select **Look at Your Preceptor's Evaluation**. Then click on **Medication Scorecard** inside the box with Dorothy Grant's name (see example on the following page).

■ MEDICATION SCORECARD

- First, review Table A. Was betamethasone given correctly? Did you give the other medications as ordered?
- Table B shows you which (if any) medications you gave incorrectly.
- Table C addresses the resources used for Dorothy Grant. Did you access the patient's chart, MAR, EPR, or Kardex as needed to make safe medication administration decisions?
- Did you check the patient's armband to verify her identity? Did you check whether your patient had any known allergies to medications? Were vital signs taken?

When you have finished reviewing the scorecard, click **Return to Evaluations** and then **Return to Menu**.

■ VITAL SIGNS

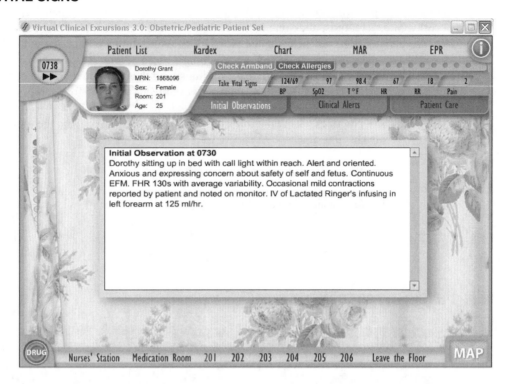

Vital signs, often considered the traditional "signs of life," include body temperature, heart rate, respiratory rate, blood pressure, oxygen saturation of the blood, and pain level.

Inside Dorothy Grant's room, click **Take Vital Signs**. (*Note:* If you are following this detailed tour step by step, you will need to **Restart the Program** from the Floor Menu, sign in again, and navigate to Room 201.) Collect vital signs for this patient and record them below. Note the time at which you collected each of these data. (*Remember:* You can take vital signs at any time. The data change over time to reflect the temporal changes you would find in a patient similar to Dorothy Grant.)

Vital Signs	Findings/Time
Blood pressure	
O$_2$ saturation	
Heart rate	
Respiratory rate	
Temperature	
Pain rating	

After you are done, click on the **EPR** icon located in the tool bar at the top of the screen. Your username and password are automatically provided. Click on **Login** to enter the EPR. To access Dorothy Grant's records, click on the down arrow next to Patient and choose her room number, **201**. Select **Vital Signs** as the category. Next, in the empty time column on the far right, record the vital signs data you just collected in the patient's room. (*Note:* If you need help with this process, see page 16.) Now compare these findings with the data you collected earlier for this patient's vital signs. Use these earlier findings to establish a baseline for each of the vital signs.

a. Are any of the data you collected significantly different from the baseline for a particular vital sign?

Circle One: Yes   No

b. If "Yes," which data are different?

■ PHYSICAL ASSESSMENT

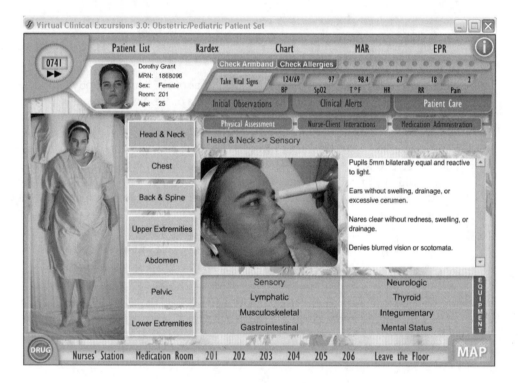

After you have finished examining the EPR for vital signs, click **Exit EPR** to return to Room 201. Click **Patient Care** and then **Physical Assessment**. Think about the information you received in the report at the beginning of this shift, as well as what you may have learned about this patient from the chart. Based on this, what area(s) of examination should you pay most attention to at this time? Is there any equipment you should be monitoring? Conduct a physical assessment of the body areas and systems that you consider priorities for Dorothy Grant. For example, select **Head & Neck**; then click on and assess **Sensory** and **Lymphatic**. Complete any other assessment(s) you think are necessary at this time. In the following table, record the data you collected during this examination.

Area of Examination	Findings
Head & Neck Sensory	
Head & Neck Lymphatic	

After you have finished collecting these data, return to the EPR. Compare the data that were already in the record with those you just collected.

    a.   Are any of the data you collected significantly different from the baselines for this patient?

       Circle One: Yes   No

    b.   If "Yes," which data are different?

■ NURSE-CLIENT INTERACTIONS

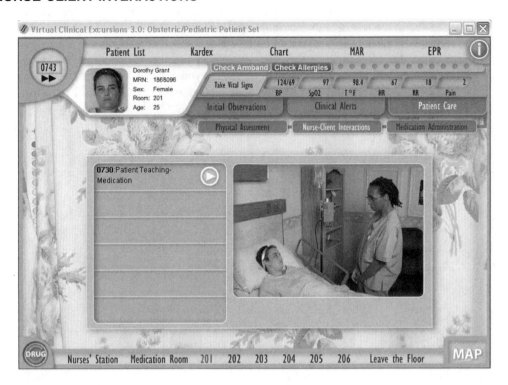

Click on **Patient Care** from inside Dorothy Grant's room (201). Now click on **Nurse-Client Interactions** to access a short video titled **Patient Teaching—Medication**, which is available for viewing at or after 0730 (based on the virtual clock in the upper left corner of your screen; see *Note* below). To begin the video, click on the white arrow next to its title. You will observe a nurse communicating with Dorothy Grant. There are many variations of nursing practice, some exemplifying "best" practice and some not. Note whether the nurse in this interaction displays professional behavior and compassionate care. Are her words congruent with what is going on with the patient? Does this interaction "feel right" to you? If not, how would you handle this situation differently? Explain.

Note: If the video you wish to view is not listed, this means you have not yet reached the correct virtual time to view that video. Check the virtual clock; you may return to access the video once its designated time has occurred—as long as you do so within the same period of care. Or you can click on the fast-forward icon within the virtual clock to advance the time by 2-minute intervals. You will then need to click again on **Patient Care** and **Nurse-Client Interactions** to refresh the screen.

At least one Nurse-Client Interactions video is available during each period of care. Viewing these videos can help you learn more about what is occurring with a patient at a certain time and also prompt you to discern between nurse communications that are ideal and those that need improvement. Compassionate care and the ability to communicate clearly are essential components of delivering quality nursing care, and it is during your clinical time that you will begin to refine these skills.

■ COLLECTING AND EVALUATING DATA

Each of the activities you perform in the Patient Care environment generates a significant amount of assessment data. Remember that after you collect data, you can record your findings in the EPR. You can also review the EPR, patient's chart, videos, and MAR at any time. You will get plenty of practice collecting and then evaluating data in context of the patient's course.

Now, here's an important question for you:

> Did the previous sequence of exercises provide the most efficient way to assess Dorothy Grant?

For example, you went to the patient's room to get vital signs, then back to the EPR to enter data and compare your findings with extant data. Next, you went back to the patient's room to do a physical examination, then again back to the EPR to enter and review data. If this back-and-forth process of data collection and recording seemed inefficient, remember the following:

- Plan all of your nursing activities to maximize efficiency, while at the same time optimizing the quality of patient care. (Think about what data you might need before performing certain tasks. For example, do you need to check a heart rate before administering a cardiac medication or check an IV site before starting an infusion?)

- You collect a tremendous amount of data when you work with a patient. Very few people can accurately remember all these data for more than a few minutes. Develop efficient assessment skills, and record data as soon as possible after collecting them.

- Assessment data are only the starting point for the nursing process.

Make a clear distinction between these first exercises and how you actually provide nursing care. These initial exercises were designed to involve you actively in the use of different software components. This workbook focuses on sensible practices for implementing the nursing process in ways that ensure the highest-quality care of patients.

Most important, remember that a human being changes through time, and that these changes include both the physical and psychosocial facets of a person as a living organism. Think about this for a moment. Some patients may change physically in a very short time (a patient with emerging myocardial infarction) or more slowly (a patient with a chronic illness). Patients' overall physical and psychosocial conditions may improve or deteriorate. They may have effective coping skills and familial support, or they may feel alone and full of despair. In fact, each individual is a complex mix of physical and psychosocial elements, and at least some of these elements usually change through time.

Thus it is crucial that you *DO NOT* think of the nursing process as a simple one-time, five-step procedure consisting of assessment, nursing diagnosis, planning, implementation, and evaluation. Rather, the nursing process should be utilized as a creative and systematic approach to delivering nursing care. Furthermore, because all living organisms are constantly changing, we must apply the nursing process over and over. Each time we follow the nursing process for an individual patient, we refine our understanding of that patient's physical and psychosocial conditions based on collection and analysis of many different types of data. *Virtual Clinical Excursions—Obstetrics-Pediatrics* will help you develop both the creativity and the systematic approach needed to become a nurse who is equipped to deliver the highest-quality care to all patients.

REDUCING MEDICATION ERRORS

Earlier in this detailed tour, you learned the basic steps of medication preparation and administration. The following simulations will allow you to practice those skills further—with an increased emphasis on reducing medication errors by using the Medication Scorecard to evaluate your work.

Sign in to work on the Obstetrics Floor at Pacific View Regional Hospital for Period of Care 1. (*Note:* If you are already working with another patient or during another period of care, click on **Leave the Floor** and then **Restart the Program**; then sign in.)

From the Patient List, select Dorothy Grant. Then click on **Go to Nurses' Station**. Complete the following steps to prepare and administer medications to Dorothy Grant.

- Click on **Medication Room**.
- Click on **MAR** and then on tab **201** to determine prn medications that have been ordered for Dorothy Grant. (*Note:* You may click on **Review MAR** at any time to verify the correct medication order. Always remember to check the patient name on the MAR to make sure you have the correct patient's record—you must click on the correct room number tab within the MAR.) Click on **Return to Medication Room** after reviewing the correct MAR.
- Click on **Unit Dosage** (or on the Unit Dosage cabinet); from the close-up view, click on drawer **201**.
- Select the medications you would like to administer. After each selection, click **Put Medication on Tray**. When you are finished selecting medications, click **Close Drawer** and then **View Medication Room**.
- Click **Automated System** (or on the Automated System unit itself). Click **Login**.
- On the next screen, specify the correct patient and drawer location.
- Select the medication you would like to administer and click **Put Medication on Tray**. Repeat this process if you wish to administer other medications from the Automated System.
- When you are finished, click **Close Drawer** and **View Medication Room**.
- From the Medication Room, click **Preparation** (or on the preparation tray).
- From the list of medications on your tray, highlight the correct medication to administer and click **Prepare**.
- This activates the Preparation Wizard. Supply any requested information; then click **Next**.
- Now select the correct patient to receive this medication and click **Finish**.
- Repeat the previous three steps until all medications that you want to administer are prepared.
- You can click on **Review Your Medications** and then on **Return to Medication Room** when ready. Once you are back in the Medication Room, go directly to Dorothy Grant's room by clicking on **201** at the bottom of the screen.
- Inside the patient's room, administer the medication, utilizing the five rights of medication administration. After you have collected the appropriate assessment data and are ready for administration, click **Patient Care** and then **Medication Administration**. Verify that the correct patient and medication(s) appear in the left-hand window. Highlight the first medication you wish to administer; then click the down arrow next to Select. From the drop-down menu, select **Administer** and complete the Administration Wizard by providing any information requested. When the Wizard stops asking for information, click **Administer to Patient**. Specify **Yes** when asked whether this administration should be recorded in the MAR. Finally, click **Finish**.

■ **SELF-EVALUATION**

Now let's see how you did during your medication administration!

- Click on **Leave the Floor** at the bottom of your screen. From the Floor Menu, select **Look at Your Preceptor's Evaluation**. Then click **Medication Scorecard**.

The following exercises will help you identify medication errors, investigate possible reasons for these errors, and reduce or prevent medication errors in the future.

1. Start by examining Table A. These are the medications you should have given to Dorothy Grant during this period of care. If each of the medications in Table A has a ✓ by it, then you made no errors. Congratulations!

If any medication has an X by it, then you made one or more medication errors.

Compare Tables A and B to determine which of the following types of errors you made: Wrong Dose, Wrong Route/Method/Site, or Wrong Time. Follow these steps:
   a. Find medications in Table A that were given incorrectly.
   b. Now see if those same medications are in Table B, which shows what you actually administered to Dorothy Grant.
   c. Comparing Tables A and B, match the Strength, Dose, Route/Method/Site, and Time for each medication you administered incorrectly.
   d. Then, using the form below, list the medications given incorrectly and mark the errors you made for each medication.

Medication	Strength	Dosage	Route	Method	Site	Time
	❏	❏	❏	❏	❏	❏
	❏	❏	❏	❏	❏	❏
	❏	❏	❏	❏	❏	❏
	❏	❏	❏	❏	❏	❏

2. To help you reduce future medication errors, consider the following list of possible reasons for errors.

- Did not check drug against MAR for correct patient, correct date, correct time, correct drug, and correct dose.
- Did not check drug dose against MAR three times.
- Did not open the unit dose package in the patient's room.
- Did not correctly identify the patient using two identifiers.
- Did not administer the drug on time.
- Did not verify patient allergies.
- Did not check the patient's current condition or vital sign parameters.
- Did not consider why the patient would be receiving this drug.
- Did not question why the drug was in the patient's drawer.
- Did not check the physician's order and/or check with the pharmacist when there was a question about the drug or dose.
- Did not verify that no adverse effects had occurred from a previous dose.

Based on the list of possibilities you just reviewed, determine how you made each error and record the reason in the form below:

Medication	Reason for Error

3. Look again at Table B. Are there medications listed that are not in Table A? If so, you gave a medication to Dorothy Grant that she should not have received. Complete the following exercises to help you understand how such an error might have been made.

a. Perhaps you gave a medication that was on Dorothy Grant's MAR for this period of care, without recognizing that a change had occurred in the patient's condition, which should have caused you to reconsider. Review patient records as necessary and complete the following form:

Medication	Possible Reasons Not to Give This Medication

b. Another possibility is that you gave Dorothy Grant a medication that should have been given at a different time. Check her MAR and complete the form below to determine whether you made a Wrong Time error:

Medication	Given to Dorothy Grant at What Time	Should Have Been Given at What Time

c. Maybe you gave another patient's medication to Dorothy Grant. In this case, you made a Wrong Patient error. Check the MARs of other patients and use the form below to determine whether you made this type of error:

Medication	Given to Dorothy Grant	Should Have Been Given to

4. The Medication Scorecard provides some other interesting sources of information. For example, if there is a medication selected for Dorothy Grant but it was not given to her, there will be an X by that medication in Table A, but it will not appear in Table B. In that case, you might have given this medication to some other patient, which is another type of Wrong Patient error. To investigate further, look at Table D, which lists the medications you gave to other patients. See whether you can find any medications ordered for Dorothy Grant that were given to another patient by mistake. However, before you make any decisions, be sure to cross-check the MAR for other patients because the same medication may have been ordered for multiple patients. Use the following form to record your findings:

Medication	Should Have Been Given to Dorothy Grant	Given by Mistake to

5. Now take some time to review the medication exercises you just completed. Use the form below to create an overall analysis of what you have learned. Once again, record each of the medication errors you made, including the type of each error. Then, for each error you made, indicate specifically what you would do differently to prevent this type of error from occurring again.

Medication	Type of Error	Error Prevention Tactic

Submit this form to your instructor if required as a graded assignment, or simply use these exercises to improve your understanding of medication errors and how to reduce them.

Name: _____   Date: _____

The following icons are used throughout this workbook to help you quickly identify particular activities and assignments:

 Indicates a reading assignment—tells you which textbook chapter(s) you should read before starting each lesson

 Indicates a writing activity

 Marks the beginning of an interactive CD-ROM activity—signals you to open or return to your *Virtual Clinical Excursions—Obstetrics-Pediatrics* CD-ROM

 Indicates additional CD-ROM instructions

 Indicates questions and activities that require you to consult your textbook

 Indicates the approximate time required to complete an exercise

High-Risk Pregnancy Assessment, Including Nutrition and Prenatal Care

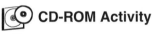 **Reading Assignment:** Prenatal Care and Adaptations to Pregnancy (Chapter 4)
Nursing Care of Women with Complications During Pregnancy
(Chapter 5)

Patients: Kelly Brady, Obstetrics Floor, Room 203
Maggie Gardner, Obstetrics Floor, Room 204

Objectives:

- Identify appropriate interventions for maintaining adequate maternal and fetal nutrition.
- Differentiate among the various types of assessment techniques that can be used with low- and high-risk pregnancy patients.
- Identify various methods of testing that can be used in high-risk pregnancies.

Exercise 1

 CD-ROM Activity

30 minutes

1. A high-risk pregnancy is one in which the health of the _____ or

   _____ is in _____.

 2. List several characteristics and causes of high-risk pregnancies. (*Hint:* Review page 78 in the textbook.)

3. What are the two types of ultrasound?

→ • Sign in to work at Pacific View Regional Hospital on the Obstetrics Floor for Period of Care 3. (*Note:* If you are already in the virtual hospital from a previous exercise, click on **Leave the Floor** and then **Restart the Program** to get to the sign-in window.)
  • From the Patient List, select Maggie Gardner (Room 204).
  • Click on **Go to Nurses' Station**.
  • Click on **Chart** and then on **204** to view Maggie Gardner's chart.
  • Click on the **Diagnostic Reports** tab and review the information given.

4. What type of ultrasound is Maggie Gardner having?

5. Based on the ultrasound findings, how large is the baby?

6. List three abnormalities found on Maggie Gardner's ultrasound in regard to the placenta.

7. What is the impression from Maggie Gardner's ultrasound in terms of the fetus and the placenta?

8. What are the recommendations regarding follow-up?

Exercise 2

 CD-ROM Activity

 30 minutes

 Read about biophysical profiles on page 81 in your textbook.

1. Biophysical profile is another very important assessment tool used with patients who are experiencing a high-risk pregnancy. What five items are assessed on a biophysical profile?

2. Biophysical profile is used to identify reduced fetal _____ in conditions associated with poor _____ function.

3. As fetal hypoxia increases, fetal heart rate changes occur first, followed by cessation of

   _____ movements,

   _____ movements, and loss of

   _____.

4. Amniotic fluid volume is _____ when placental function is poor.

→ • Sign in to work at Pacific View Regional Hospital on the Obstetrics Floor for Period of Care 3. (*Note:* If you are already in the virtual hospital from a previous exercise, click on **Leave the Floor** and then **Restart the Program** to get to the sign-in window.)
   • From the Patient List, select Kelly Brady (Room 203).
   • Click on **Go to Nurses' Station**.
   • Click on **Chart** and then on **203** to view Kelly Brady's chart.
   • Click on the **Diagnostic Reports** tab and review the information given.

5. What is the estimated gestational age of Kelly Brady's fetus?

6. What is the amniotic fluid index as indicated on the report?

7. If there were an abnormal amniotic fluid index on Kelly Brady's report, what might that indicate?

8. What is the normal size of a pocket of amniotic fluid?

9. What measurement would indicate oligohydramnios? Polyhydramnios?

Exercise 3

 CD-ROM Activity

 30 minutes

- Sign in to work at Pacific View Regional Hospital on the Obstetrics Floor for Period of Care 1. (*Note:* If you are already in the virtual hospital from a previous exercise, click on **Leave the Floor** and then **Restart the Program** to get to the sign-in window.)
- From the Patient List, select Maggie Gardner (Room 204).
- Click on **Go to Nurses' Station**.
- Click on **Chart** and then on **204** to view Maggie Gardner's chart.
- Click on the **Laboratory Reports** tab and review the information given.

 Review information regarding anemia on pages 60-61 and 103-104 in your textbook.

1. What are Maggie Gardner's hemoglobin and hematocrit levels?

 • Click on the **History and Physical** tab in Maggie Gardner's chart.

2. What puts Maggie Gardner at a greater risk for developing anemia than the average pregnancy patient? (*Hint:* Review the Genetic Screening section of her History and Physical.)

3. What is the recommended daily amount of iron for nonpregnant women? For pregnant women?

4. What is a normal hemoglobin level for a woman who is pregnant?

5. What assessments specifically related to an anemia diagnosis need to be performed by the nurse at each visit?

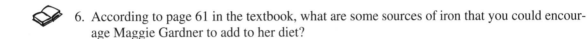

6. According to page 61 in the textbook, what are some sources of iron that you could encourage Maggie Gardner to add to her diet?

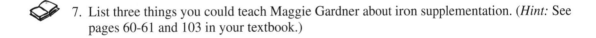

7. List three things you could teach Maggie Gardner about iron supplementation. (*Hint:* See pages 60-61 and 103 in your textbook.)

Nursing Care of Women with Complications During Pregnancy: Antepartal Bleeding Disorders

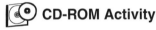 **Reading Assignment:** Nursing Care of Women with Complications During Pregnancy
(Chapter 5, pages 89-90)

Patient: Gabriela Valenzuela, Obstetrics Floor, Room 205

Objectives:

- Identify appropriate interventions for managing abruptio placenta.
- Differentiate between the symptoms of abruptio placenta and those of placenta previa.
- Plan and evaluate essential patient education during the acute phase of diagnosis.

Exercise 1

 CD-ROM Activity

30 minutes

- Sign in to work at Pacific View Regional Hospital on the Obstetrics Floor for Period of Care 1. (*Note:* If you are already in the virtual hospital from a previous exercise, click on **Leave the Floor** and then **Restart the Program** to get to the sign-in window.)
- From the Patient List, select Gabriela Valenzuela (Room 205).
- Click on **Go to Nurses' Station**.
- Click on **Chart** and then on **205**.
- Click on the **Emergency Department** tab and review the information given.

1. What brought Gabriela Valenzuela to the Emergency Department? How long did she wait to come to the ED, and what was the deciding factor in her coming to the ED?

49

Read about the incidence and etiology of abruptio placenta on page 89 in your textbook.

2. Other than a motor vehicle accident, what could result in or increase the risk for having an abruptio placenta?

 3. Differential diagnosis is very important when a patient presents with clinical manifestations that could be evidence of more than one process. Complete the following table by comparing abruptio placenta and placenta previa. (*Hint:* Refer to Table 5-5 on page 88 in your textbook for help.)

Characteristic/ Complication	Abruptio Placenta	Placenta Previa
Bleeding		
Shock complication		
Blood clotting		
Uterine tonicity		
Tenderness/pain		
Placenta findings		
Fetal		

4. Based on your review of the ED record, what type of abruption does Gabriela Valenzuela have? Provide supporting documentation from the notes in the ED record. (*Hint:* Review Table 5-5 on page 88 in your textbook).

 • Click on **Return to Nurses' Station** and then on **205** to go to the patient's room.
   • Inside the room, click on **Patient Care** and then on **Nurse-Client Interactions**.
   • Select and view the video titled **0740: Patient Teaching—Fetal Monitor**. (*Note:* Check the virtual clock to see whether enough time has elapsed. You can use the fast-forward feature to advance the time by 2-minute intervals if the video is not yet available. Then click again on **Patient Care** and **Nurse-Client Interactions** to refresh the screen.)

   5. Once Gabriela Valenzuela is admitted to the floor, what are her and her husband's concerns? What does the nurse include in her teaching to alleviate those concerns?

 • Again, click on **Patient Care** and then on **Nurse-Client Interactions**.
   • Select and view the video titled **0805: Abruption**. (*Note:* Check the virtual clock to see whether enough time has elapsed. You can use the fast-forward feature to advance the time by 2-minute intervals if the video is not yet available. Then click again on **Patient Care** and **Nurse-Client Interactions** to refresh the screen.)

   6. What interventions will help to increase the oxygen supply to the baby and prevent further separation of the placenta?

Exercise 2

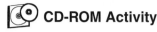 **CD-ROM Activity**

 20 minutes

- Sign in to work at Pacific View Regional Hospital on the Obstetrics Floor for Period of Care 1. (*Note:* If you are already in the virtual hospital from a previous exercise, click on **Leave the Floor** and then **Restart the Program** to get to the sign-in window.)
- From the Patient List, select Gabriela Valenzuela (Room 205).
- Click on **Go to Nurses' Station**.

Gabriela Valenzuela is at increased risk for early delivery as a result of her earlier abdominal trauma and the subsequent occurrence of a grade 1 abruptio placenta. She is currently manifesting signs and symptoms of early labor. According to the Emergency Department notes, she was given a dose of betamethasone, which was to be repeated in 12 hours.

 1. What is the purpose of the administration of betamethasone in Gabriela Valenzuela's situation? (*Hint:* See page 193 in your textbook.)

 - Click on **MAR** and then on tab **205**.
- Review the dosage of betamethasone to be given.
- Click on **Return to Nurses' Station** and then on **Medication Room**.
- Click on **Unit Dosage** and then on drawer **205**.
- Click on **Betamethasone**; then click **Put Medication on Tray**.
- Click on **Close Drawer**.
- Click on **View Medication Room** and then on **Preparation**.
- Click on **Prepare** and follow the prompts of the Preparation Wizard.
- Click on **Return to Medication Room** and then on **205** to return to the patient's room.
- Inside the room, click on **Patient Care** and then on **Medication Administration**.
- Click on **Review Your Medications** and then click on the **Prepared** tab.

2. According to the box on the right side of your screen, what is the medication name and dosage that you have prepared for Gabriela Valenzuela?

3. Based on your answer to question 2, how many mg are you giving to Gabriela Valenzuela? Is this the correct dosage based on the MAR?

• Click on **Return to Room 205**.
   • Click on the **Drug** icon in left-hand corner of your screen.
   • Use the search box or scroll down the list of medications to find betamethasone.

4. Based on the information provided in the Drug Guide, what is the indication and dosage of betamethasone for pregnant adults?

5. After reviewing the baseline assessment data in the Drug Guide, what areas need to be assessed in Gabriela Valenzuela's history?

6. Review the information regarding the administration of betamethasone. What are three things that must be taken into consideration when giving this medication in the injection form?

7. What are the five rights of medication administration?

   (1)

   (2)

   (3)

   (4)

   (5)

Now you are ready to complete the medication administration.

• Click on **Return to Room 205**.
   • Click on **Check Armband**.
   • Click on **Patient Care** and then on **Medication Administration**.
   • View medications set aside for Gabriela Valenzuela.
   • Follow the prompts to administer Gabriela Valenzuela's betamethasone.
   • Document the injection in the MAR.
   • Click on **Leave the Floor** and then on **Look at Your Preceptor's Evaluation**.
   • Click on **Medication Scorecard**. How did you do?

Exercise 3

 CD-ROM Activity

20 minutes

- Sign in to work at Pacific View Regional Hospital on the Obstetrics Floor for Period of Care 2. (*Note:* If you are already in the virtual hospital from a previous exercise, click on **Leave the Floor** and then **Restart the Program** to get to the sign-in window.)
- From the Patient List, select Gabriela Valenzuela (Room 205).
- Click on **Go to Nurses' Station**.
- Click on **Chart** and then on **205**.
- Click on the **Diagnostic Reports** tab and review the information given.

1. Gabriela Valenzuela had an ultrasound on Tuesday to determine the source of her bleeding. What were the findings of the ultrasound?

→ • Click on the **Laboratory Reports** tab and review the results.

2. What are Gabriela Valenzuela's hemoglobin and hematocrit levels on Tuesday? How does this compare with Wednesday's report? Is there a significant change?

 3. According to the textbook, the hematocrit level needs to be maintained between _____ and _____%. (*Hint:* See page 52 in your textbook.)

Review page 89 in your textbook.

4. What clinical manifestations would indicate that there is a worsening in the condition of either the patient or the fetus?

→ • Click on **Return to Nurses' Station**.
- Click on **EPR** and then on **Login**.
- Select **205** for the patient's room.
- Using the right and left arrows, scroll to review vital signs over the last 12 hours.

5. Based on her vital signs from 0000 Wednesday until 1200 on Wednesday, would you consider Gabriela Valenzuela's condition stable or unstable? What is your rationale?

- Click on **Exit EPR**.
- Click on **205** at the bottom of the screen.
- Click on **Patient Care** and then on **Nurse-Client Interactions**.
- Select and view the video titled **1140: Intervention—Bleeding, Comfort**. Take notes regarding the interaction. (*Note:* Check the virtual clock to see whether enough time has elapsed. You can use the fast-forward feature to advance the time by 2-minute intervals if the video is not yet available. Then click again on **Patient Care** and **Nurse-Client Interactions** to refresh the screen.)

6. What happened that elicited this interaction? (*Hint:* In the patient's chart, review the Nurse's Notes for 1140.)

7. What actions did the nurse take during the interaction with the patient? (Include what is documented in the Nurse's Notes.)

Exercise 4

 CD-ROM Activity

 20 minutes

- Sign in to work at Pacific View Regional Hospital on the Obstetrics Floor for Period of Care 3. (*Note:* If you are already in the virtual hospital from a previous exercise, click on **Leave the Floor** and then **Restart the Program** to get to the sign-in window.)
- From the Patient List, select Gabriela Valenzuela (Room 205).
- Click on **Go to Nurses' Station**.
- Click on **Kardex** and then on tab **205**.

1. What problem areas related to Gabriela Valenzuela's diagnosis have been identified by the nurse?

2. What is the focus of the expected outcomes related to these problems?

3. Using standard NANDA nursing diagnosis wording and format, write four possible nursing diagnoses for Gabriela Valenzuela.

→ • Click on **Return to Nurses' Station**.
  • Click on **Chart** and then on **205**.
  • Click on the **Patient Education** tab and review the information given.

4. According to the patient education sheet in Gabriela Valenzuela's chart, what are the educational goals related to her diagnosis?

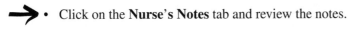 • Click on the **Nurse's Notes** tab and review the notes.

5. What patient education has been completed by the nurses from Gabriela Valenzuela's admission through Period of Care 3? Include documentation of times and topics.

6. What are some barriers to learning that the nurse may confront with Gabriela Valenzuela? (*Hint:* Review the Nurse's Notes in the chart.)

7. How can the nurse overcome each of these barriers?

Nursing Care of Women with Complications During Pregnancy: Gestational Hypertension

/✺ **Reading Assignment:** Nursing Care of Women with Complications During Pregnancy
(Chapter 5, pages 90-94)

Patient: Kelly Brady, Obstetrics Floor, Room 203

Objectives:

- Assess and identify signs and symptoms present in the patient with severe preeclampsia.
- Explain how common signs and symptoms present in the patient with severe preeclampsia relate to the underlying pathophysiology of this disease.
- Identify the patient who has developed HELLP syndrome.
- Describe routine nursing care for the patient with severe preeclampsia who is receiving magnesium sulfate.

In this lesson you will assess and plan care for a patient with severe preeclampsia who then develops HELLP syndrome and delivers at 26²/₇ weeks gestation.

Exercise 1

 CD-ROM Activity

 30 minutes

- Sign in to work at Pacific View Regional Hospital on the Obstetrics Floor for Period of Care 3. (*Note:* If you are already in the virtual hospital from a previous exercise, click on **Leave the Floor** and then **Restart the Program** to get to the sign-in window.)
- From the Patient List, select Kelly Brady (Room 203).
- Click on **Go to Nurses' Station**.
- Click on **Chart** and then on **203**.
- Click on the **History and Physical** tab and review the information given.

1. What was Kelly Brady's diagnosis on admission?

2. Using the History and Physical and pages 90-91 in your textbook, complete the table below.

Sign/ Symptom	Gestational Hypertension	Severe Preeclampsia	Kelly Brady on Admission
Blood pressure			
Proteinuria			
Headache			
Reflexes			
Visual problems			
Epigastric pain			
Edema			

• Click on the **Physician's Orders** tab and find the admitting physician's orders on Tuesday at 1030.

3. What tests/procedures did Kelly Brady's physician order to confirm the diagnosis of severe preeclampsia?

 • Click on the **Physician's Notes** tab and review the note for Wednesday 0730.

4. What subjective and objective data are recorded here that would support the diagnosis of severe preeclampsia?

• Kelly Brady's 24-hour urine collection was completed and sent to the lab at 1230.
• Click on the **Laboratory Reports** tab and review the results for Wednesday 1230.

5. What were the results of Kelly Brady's 24-hour urine collection?

6. Now list all the data you have collected during this exercise that confirm Kelly Brady's diagnosis of severe preeclampsia.

Exercise 2

 CD-ROM Activity

 30 minutes

• Sign in to work at Pacific View Regional Hospital on the Obstetrics Floor for Period of Care 1. (*Note:* If you are already in the virtual hospital from a previous exercise, click on **Leave the Floor** and then **Restart the Program** to get to the sign-in window.)
• From the Patient List, select Kelly Brady (Room 203).
• Click on **Go to Nurses' Station** and then on **203**.
• Click on **Take Vital Signs**.

1. Record Kelly Brady's current vital signs below. (*Note:* Answers will vary depending on the exact time you take them.)

Temperature:

Heart Rate:

Respirations:

Blood Pressure:

Pain Rating:

→ • Click **Patient Care** and perform a physical assessment by selecting the various body areas (yellow buttons) and system subcategories (green buttons) as specified in the table in question 2.

2. Record your findings from the focused assessment of Kelly Brady in the table below.

Assessment Area	Kelly Brady's Findings
Head & Neck Sensory	
Neurologic	
Chest Respiratory	
Abdomen Gastrointestinal	
Lower Extremities Neurologic	

Read pages 91-92 in your textbook before answering the following questions.

3. The main pathogenic factor present in the woman with gestational hypertension is

_____ leading to a _____ in blood flow to all mother's

organs and _____, resulting in _____,

_____, and _____.

4. Match each sign or symptom below with the preeclampsia-associated pathology it indicates. (*Note:* Some letters will be used more than once.)

Sign/Symptom	**Pathology**
_____ Blurred vision/blind spots	a. Generalized vasoconstriction
_____ Headache	b. Glomerular damage
_____ Epigastric or right upper quadrant abdominal pain	c. Retinal arteriolar spasms
_____ Hyperreflexia	d. Hepatic microemboli; liver damage
_____ Elevated blood pressure	e. Cortical brain spasms
_____ Proteinuria/oliguria	

Exercise 3

 CD-ROM Activity

 30 minutes

- Sign in to work at Pacific View Regional Hospital on the Obstetrics Floor for Period of Care 3. (*Note:* If you are already in the virtual hospital from a previous exercise, click on **Leave the Floor** and then **Restart the Program** to get to the sign-in window.)
- From the Patient List, select Kelly Brady (Room 203).
- Click on **Go to Nurses' Station**.

 Read about HELLP syndrome on page 91 in your textbook.

1. Why do you think Kelly Brady had blood drawn at 1230 for an AST measurement and a platelet count?

➤ • Click on **Chart** and then on **203**.
  • Click on the **Laboratory Reports** tab and review the results for Wednesday 1230.

  2. Complete the table below based on your review of the Laboratory Reports and your textbook reading.

Test	Wednesday 1230 Result	Value in HELLP
Platelet count		
AST		

➤ • Click on **Return to Nurses' Station** and then on Patient List.
  • Click on **Get Report** for Kelly Brady.

  3. Why has Kelly Brady been transferred to Labor and Delivery?

  4. HELLP syndrome is not a separate illness but a variant of _____.

     HELLP syndrome consists of intravascular _____, elevated

     _____, and low _____.

➤ • Click on **Return to Nurses' Station**.
  • Click on **Chart** and then on **203**.
  • Click on the **Physician's Notes** tab and review the note for Wednesday 1530.

  5. What is the physician's plan of care for Kelly Brady in light of the HELLP syndrome diagnosis?

You will be the nurse caring for Kelly Brady after her surgery while she is receiving magnesium sulfate. Read about this medication on page 92 in your textbook.

6. All of the assessments/interventions listed below are part of routine nursing care for a patient with severe preeclampsia. Place an X beside each of the activities performed specifically to assess for magnesium toxicity.

_____ a. Measure/record urine output.

_____ b. Measure proteinuria using urine dipstick.

_____ c. Monitor liver enzyme levels and platelet count.

_____ d. Monitor for headache, visual disturbances, and epigastric pain.

_____ e. Assess for decreased level of consciousness.

_____ f. Assess DTRs.

_____ g. Weigh daily to assess for edema

_____ h. Monitor vital signs, especially respiratory rate.

_____ i. Dim room lights and maintain a quiet environment.

LESSON 4

Nursing Care of Women with Complications During Pregnancy: Gestational Diabetes Mellitus (GDM)

Reading Assignment: Nursing Care of Women with Complications During Pregnancy
(Chapter 5, pages 96-102)

Patient: Stacey Crider, Obstetrics Floor, Room 202

Objectives:

- Identify appropriate interventions for controlling hyperglycemia in a patient with gestational diabetes mellitus (GDM).
- Correctly administer insulin to a patient with GDM.
- Plan and evaluate essential patient teaching for a patient with GDM.

In this lesson you will describe, plan, and evaluate the care of a patient with GDM.

Exercise 1

 CD-ROM Activity

 30 minutes

 Read about pain and the interventions used to relieve pain on pages 588-589 in your textbook.

- Sign in to work at Pacific View Regional Hospital on the Obstetrics Floor for Period of Care 2. (*Note:* If you are already in the virtual hospital from a previous exercise, click on **Leave the Floor** and then **Restart the Program** to get to the sign-in window.)
- From the Patient List, select Stacey Crider (Room 202).
- Click on **Go to Nurses' Station**.
- Click on **Chart** and then on **202**.
- Click on the **History and Physical** tab and review the information given.

1. When was Stacey Crider's GDM diagnosed? How has it been managed so far?

2. List the risk factors for GDM. (*Hint:* See page 92 in your textbook.)

➡ • Click on the **Nursing Admission** tab and review the information given.

3. Search for evidence of risk factors for GDM in the History and Physical and Nursing Admission sections of Stacey Crider's chart. What risk factors are present?

4. What does Stacey Crider's physician suspect is the cause of her poorly controlled blood glucose levels? (*Hint:* See the physician's impression within her History and Physical.)

➡ • Click on the **Physician's Orders** tab.

5. Review Stacey Crider's admission orders and list the orders that are related to her GDM.

6. Why did Stacey Crider's physician order a hemoglobin A1C test as part of her admission labs? (*Hint:* See page 100 in your textbook.)

 • Click on **Return to Nurses' Station**.
 • Click on the **Drug** icon in the lower left corner of the screen.
 • Use the search box or scroll down the list of medications to find betamethasone.

7. On admission, Stacey Crider was in preterm labor. This was treated with magnesium sulfate tocolysis. She was also given a course of betamethasone. How might betamethasone affect her GDM?

 • Click on **Return to Nurses' Station**.
 • Click on **Chart** and then on **202**.
 • Click on the **Physician's Notes** tab and review the note for Tuesday at 0700.

8. How does Stacey Crider's physician plan to deal with these potential medication effects?

 • Click on **Return to Nurses' Station** and then on **202**.
 • Click on **Patient Care** and then on **Nurse-Client Interactions**.
 • Select and view the video titled **1115: Teaching—Diet, Infection**. (*Note:* Check the virtual clock to see whether enough time has elapsed. You can use the fast-forward feature to advance the time by 2-minute intervals if the video is not yet available. Then click again on **Patient Care** and **Nurse-Client Interactions** to refresh the screen.)

9. Stacey Crider's other admission diagnosis is bacterial vaginosis (BV). What is the relationship between the bacterial vaginosis infection and her GDM?

Exercise 2

  CD-ROM Activity

15 minutes

- Sign in to work at Pacific View Regional Hospital on the Obstetrics Floor for Period of Care 1. (*Note:* If you are already in the virtual hospital from a previous exercise, click on **Leave the Floor** and then **Restart the Program** to get to the sign-in window.)
- From the Patient List, select Stacey Crider (Room 202).
- Click on **Go to Nurses' Station**.
- Click on the **Drug** icon in the lower left corner of the screen.
- Stacey Crider needs her insulin so that she can eat breakfast. She receives lispro insulin before each meal and NPH insulin at bedtime. Read about the differences in these two types of insulin in the Drug Guide.

1. Based on the Drug Guide, complete the table below. (*Note:* NPH is considered an intermediate-acting insulin.)

Type of Insulin	Onset of Action	Peak	Duration
Lispro			
Intermediate-acting			

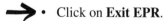 - Click on **Return to Nurses' Station**.
- Click on **EPR** and then on **Login**.
- Specify **202** as the patient's room and **Vital Signs** as the category.
- Review the vital sign assessment for Wednesday at 0700.

2. What is Stacey Crider's blood glucose?

- Click on **Exit EPR**.
- Click on **MAR** and then on **202**.

3. What is Stacey Crider's prescribed insulin dosage?

• Click on **Return to Nurses' Station**.
  • Click on **Chart** and then on **202**.
  • Click on the **Physician's Orders** tab and review the orders for Tuesday at 1900.

4. How much insulin should Stacey Crider receive? Why?

 • Click on **Return to Nurses' Station**.
  • Click on **Medication Room**.
  • Click on **Unit Dosage** and then on drawer **202**.
  • Select **Insulin lispro**; then click on **Put Medication on Tray**.
  • Click on **Close Drawer** and then on **View Medication Room**.
  • Click on **Preparation** and then on **Prepare**.
  • Follow the prompts to complete preparation of Stacey Crider's lispro insulin dose.
  • Click on **Return to Medication Room**.

You are almost ready to give Stacey Crider's insulin injection. However, before you do . . .

5. Consider lispro insulin's rapid onset of action. What else should you check before giving Stacey Crider her injection?

Now you're ready!

 • Click on **202** to return to the patient's room.
  • Inside the room, click on **Check Armband**.
  • Click on **Patient Care** and then on **Medication Administration**.
  • Insulin lispro should be listed as medication set aside for Stacey Crider.
  • Click on the arrow next to Select and choose **Administer** from the drop-down menu.
  • Follow the prompts to administer Stacey Crider's insulin injection. Document the injection in the MAR.
  • Click on **Leave the Floor**; then click **Look at Your Preceptor's Evaluation**.
  • Click on **Medication Scorecard**. How did you do?

Exercise 3

 CD-ROM Activity

 30 minutes

- Sign in to work at Pacific View Regional Hospital on the Obstetrics Floor for Period of Care 3. (*Note:* If you are already in the virtual hospital from a previous exercise, click on **Leave the Floor** and then **Restart the Program** to get to the sign-in window.)
- From the Patient List, select Stacey Crider.
- Click on **Go to Nurses' Station**.
- Click on **Chart** and then on **202**.
- Click on the **Patient Education** tab.
- Stacey Crider will probably be discharged soon. Review her Patient Education record to determine her learning needs in relation to GDM.

1. List the educational goals for Stacey Crider regarding GDM.

Read the Antepartum Care section on pages 100-101 in your textbook.

2. Which of Stacey Crider's educational goals would apply to all women with GDM?

3. Which of Stacey Crider's educational goals would not apply to all women with GDM? Support your answer.

→ • Click on the **Nurse's Notes** tab and review the note for 0600 Wednesday.

4. How did the nurse describe Stacey Crider's ability to give her own insulin injection at that time?

→ • Click again on **Patient Education**.

5. What teaching has already been done with this patient on Wednesday in regard to GDM?

→ • Click on **Nurse's Notes** and scroll to the note for 1200 Wednesday.

6. Do you think today's initial teaching on insulin administration was effective? Support your answer using objective documentation from the Nurse's Notes.

7. Stacey Crider needs to know all of the following information. Which topic(s) would you choose to work on with her during this period of care? (*Hint:* Review the Patient Education and Nurse's Notes in her chart.)

_____ a. Verbalize appropriate food choices and portions.

_____ b. Demonstrate good technique when administering insulin

_____ c. Demonstrate good technique with self-monitoring of blood glucose.

_____ d. Recognize hyper- and hypoglycemia and how to treat each.

8. Give a rationale for the choice(s) you made in the previous question.

9. Which of the following topics do you think Stacey Crider would most likely choose to work on during this period of care?
   a. Verbalize appropriate food choices and portions.
   b. Demonstrate good technique when administering insulin.
   c. Demonstrate good technique with self-monitoring of blood glucose.
   d. Recognize hyper- and hypoglycemia and how to treat each.

10. Give a rationale for the choice you made in the previous question.

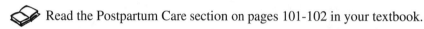 Read the Postpartum Care section on pages 101-102 in your textbook.

11. Stacey Crider has a significant risk for developing glucose intolerance later in life. What advice would you give Stacey Crider to reduce this risk?

12. Could Stacey Crider's GDM affect her baby after birth? Explain.

Nursing Care of Women with Complications During Pregnancy: Cardiac and Lupus

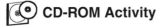 **Reading Assignment:** Nursing Care of Women with Complications During Pregnancy
(Chapter 5, pages 102-104)

Patients: Maggie Gardner, Obstetrics Floor, Room 204
Gabriela Valenzuela, Obstetrics Floor, Room 205

Objectives:

- Identify appropriate interventions for managing selected medical-surgical problems in pregnancy.
- Plan and evaluate essential patient education during the acute phase of diagnosis.

Exercise 1

 CD-ROM Activity

15 minutes

- Sign in to work at Pacific View Regional Hospital on the Obstetrics Floor for Period of Care 1. (*Note:* If you are already in the virtual hospital from a previous exercise, click on **Leave the Floor** and then **Restart the Program** to get to the sign-in window.)
- From the Patient List, select Gabriela Valenzuela (Room 205).
- Click on **Go to Nurses' Station**.
- Click on **Chart** and then on **205** to view Gabriela Valenzuela's chart.
- Click on the **History and Physical** tab and review the information given.

 Review cardiac problems during pregnancy on pages 102-103 of your textbook.

1. According to the textbook, heart disease complicates a small percentage of pregnancies. After reviewing the History and Physical for Gabriela Valenzuela, what does the physician note as her cardiac problem?

2. Cardiac failure can occur during _____ portion of pregnancy, including

   the _____ period.

3. According to the History and Physical, what cardiac symptoms does Gabriela Valenzuela exhibit now that she is pregnant?

4. Based on your reading, why do pregnant women with cardiac disorders have problems during their pregnancies?

5. What abnormal assessment finding is noted in the History and Physical that would be associated with Gabriela Valenzuela's cardiac disorder?

Exercise 2

 CD-ROM Activity

 15 minutes

- Sign in to work at Pacific View Regional Hospital on the Obstetrics Floor for Period of Care 2. (*Note:* If you are already in the virtual hospital from a previous exercise, click on **Leave the Floor** and then **Restart the Program** to get to the sign-in window.)
- From the Patient List, select Maggie Gardner (Room 204).
- Click on **Go to Nurses' Station**.
- Click on **Chart** and then on **204** to view Maggie Gardner's chart.
- Click on the **History and Physical** tab and review the information given.

Autoimmune disorders encompass a wide variety of disorders that can be disruptive to the pregnancy process. Maggie Gardner has been admitted to rule out lupus. The following questions will explore the various aspects of this autoimmune disorder. You may want to review information from a medical-surgical textbook regarding this disease.

1. What information in Maggie Gardner's History and Physical would correlate to a diagnosis of SLE?

 • Click on **Return to Nurses' Station** and then on **204** at the bottom of the screen.
• Click on **Patient Care** and complete a head-to-toe assessment of Maggie Gardner. (*Note:* Record your findings in question 2 below.)

2. List at least four abnormal findings related to Maggie Gardner's potential diagnosis.

→ • Click on **Chart** and then on **204** to view Maggie Gardner's chart.
• Click on the **Patient Education** tab and review the information given.

3. Based on your physical assessment of Maggie Gardner, the information presented in the Patient Education section of the chart, and the fact that this is a new diagnosis for the patient, list at least three areas of teaching that need to be completed for this patient.

Exercise 3

 CD-ROM Activity

 15 minutes

• Sign in to work at Pacific View Regional Hospital on the Obstetrics Floor for Period of Care 3. (*Note:* If you are already in the virtual hospital from a previous exercise, click on **Leave the Floor** and then **Restart the Program** to get to the sign-in window.)
• From the Patient List, select Maggie Gardner (Room 204).
• Click on **Go to Nurses' Station**.
• Click on **Chart** and then on **204** to view Maggie Gardner's chart.
• Click on the **Consultations** tab review the Rheumatology Consult.

1. List four things that the rheumatologist notes in his impressions regarding specific findings associated with a diagnosis of SLE.

→ • Click on the **Diagnostic Reports** tab and review the information given.

2. Maggie Gardner had an ultrasound done before the consult with the rheumatologist. What were the findings in regard to SLE? What were the follow-up recommendations? (*Hint:* See Impression section.)

3. What is the rheumatologist's plan regarding laboratory/diagnostics to gain a definitive diagnosis?

4. According to the Rheumatology Consult, what is the plan regarding medications (immediate need)?

→ • Click on **Return to Nurses' Station**.
  • Click on the **Drug** icon in the lower left corner of the screen.
  • Use the search box or scroll down the list of medications to find and review prednisone.

5. What does Maggie Gardner need to be taught regarding prednisone?

• Click on **Return to Nurse's Station** and then on **204** at the bottom of the screen.
- Click on **Patient Care** and then on **Nurse-Client Interactions**.
- Select and view the video titled **1530: Disease Management**. (*Note:* Check the virtual clock to see whether enough time has elapsed. You can use the fast-forward feature to advance the time by 2-minute intervals if the video is not yet available. Then click again on **Patient Care** and **Nurse-Client Interactions** to refresh the screen.)

6. During this video, the nurse provides Maggie Gardner with information regarding her disease. What two things does the nurse note that are important aspects of disease management during pregnancy?

7. What medication ordered by the rheumatologist will assist in the blood flow to the placenta? How does this medication achieve this effect?

8. What key component does the nurse identify for Maggie Gardner that will assist in maintaining a healthy pregnancy?

9. What does Maggie Gardner give as her reason for not keeping previous appointments? (*Hint:* See the Nursing Admission in her chart.)

Exercise 4

 CD-ROM Activity

 15 minutes

- Sign in to work at Pacific View Regional Hospital on the Obstetrics Floor for Period of Care 4. (*Note:* If you are already in the virtual hospital from a previous exercise, click on **Leave the Floor** and then **Restart the Program** to get to the sign-in window.)
- Click on **Chart** and then on **204** to view Maggie Gardner's chart. (*Remember:* You are not able to visit patients or administer medications during Period of Care 4. You are able to review patients' records only.)
- Click on the **Laboratory Reports** tab and review the results.

1. What were Maggie Gardner's results for the following laboratory tests?

Laboratory Test	Maggie Gardner's Results
C3	
C4	
CH50	
RPR	
ANA titer	
Anticardiolipin	
Anti-sm, anti-DNA, anti-SSA	
Anti-SSB	
Anti-RVV, antiphospholipid	

 • Click on the **Consultations** tab and review the Rheumatology Consult.

2. The above lab findings are definitive for the diagnosis of SLE. According to the textbook and the Rheumatology Consult, what will be the plan to manage this disease once Maggie Gardner's baby is delivered?

➜ • Click on the **Nurse's Notes** tab and review the information given.

3. Maggie Gardner has been provided with education regarding various aspects of her disease process, testing, and hospital procedures. Based on your review of the Nurse's Notes for Wednesday, list what she has been specifically taught during the four periods of care today. (*Note:* Include the time and instruction provided.)

4. Using NANDA nursing diagnosis wording and format, write three possible nursing diagnoses for Maggie Gardner.

5. SLE requires long-term management as patients experience remissions and exacerbations. What did the rheumatologist do to establish the long-term relationship necessary with Maggie Gardner to ensure a healthy outcome?

Nursing Care of Women with Complications During Pregnancy: Substance Abuse/Battering

Reading Assignment: Nursing Care of Women with Complications During Pregnancy
(Chapter 5, pages 108-112)

Patients: Dorothy Grant, Obstetrics Floor, Room 201
Laura Wilson, Obstetrics Floor, Room 206

Objectives:

- Assess and plan care for a substance-abusing woman with a term pregnancy.
- Discuss the statistics related to battering.
- List characteristics of battered women.
- Explore the myths and facts regarding battering.
- Identify the nurse's role in regard to battered women.

Exercise 1

 CD-ROM Activity

 30 minutes

- Sign in to work at Pacific View Regional Hospital on the Obstetrics Floor for Period of Care 1. (*Note:* If you are already in the virtual hospital from a previous exercise, click on **Leave the Floor** and then **Restart the Program** to get to the sign-in window.)
- From the Patient List, select Laura Wilson (Room 206).
- Click on **Go to Nurses' Station**.
- Click on **Chart** and then on **206** to view Laura Wilson's chart.
- Click on the **Nursing Admission** tab and review the information given.

1. Complete the table below with information on Laura Wilson's use of alcohol and recreational drugs. (*Hint:* See page 4 of the Nursing Admission.)

Substance	Reported Use
Tobacco	
Alcohol	
Marijuana	
Crack cocaine	

 Read about tobacco, alcohol, marijuana, and cocaine in the Substance Abuse section on pages 108-110 in your textbook.

2. Complete the table below by placing an X under each substance thought to be associated with the listed pregnancy-related risks.

Pregnancy-Related Risk	Tobacco	Alcohol	Marijuana	Cocaine
Miscarriage				
Placental perfusion abnormalities				
Preterm labor/birth				
Fetal alcohol syndrome (FAS)				
Fetal alcohol effects (FAE)				
Hypertension				
Fetal abnormalities				
Low birth weight or fetal growth restriction				
Mental retardation and/or developmental problems (child)				
Addiction in the newborn				

• Click on **Return to Nurses' Station** and then on **206** at the bottom of the screen.

• Click on **Patient Care** and then on **Nurse-Client Interactions**.

• Select and view the video titled **1115: Teaching—Effects of Drug Use**. (*Note:* Check the virtual clock to see whether enough time has elapsed. You can use the fast-forward feature to advance the time by 2-minute intervals if the video is not yet available. Then click again on **Patient Care** and **Nurse-Client Interactions** to refresh the screen.)

3. Does Laura Wilson consider herself to be addicted? Support your answer with comments from the video interaction.

4. How does Laura Wilson think her drug use will affect the baby?

5. According to the nurse in the video, how might Laura Wilson's drug use affect the baby?

6. Assume that you are the nurse caring for Laura Wilson today. Which interventions dealing with her drug use would be most appropriate at this time?

_____ a. Talk with her in a manner that conveys caring and concern.

_____ b. Urge her to begin a drug treatment program today.

_____ c. Explain to Laura Wilson that she may lose custody of her baby if her drug use continues.

_____ d. Involve other members of the health care team in Laura Wilson's care.

7. Provide rationales for the interventions you chose in the previous answer.

Exercise 2

 CD-ROM Activity

 45 minutes

 1. Battering occurs in _____ ethnic groups and at _____
social levels. (*Hint:* See pages 111-112 of the textbook.)

 • Sign in to work at Pacific View Regional Hospital on the Obstetrics Floor for Period of
Care 1. (*Note:* If you are already in the virtual hospital from a previous exercise, click on
Leave the Floor and then **Restart the Program** to get to the sign-in window.)
• From the Patient List, select Dorothy Grant (Room 201).
• Click on **Go to Nurses' Station**.
• Click on **Chart** and then on **201** to view Dorothy Grant's chart.
• Click on the **Nursing Admission** tab and review Dorothy Grant's perspective of her abusive
relationship.

 Review the characteristics of battered women found on pages 111-112 in the textbook.

2. What is the reality of Dorothy Grant's situation (as evidenced in the Nursing Admission),
and how does that correlate with the textbook reading?

 • Click on **Return to Nurses' Station** and then on **201** at the bottom of the screen.
• Click on **Patient Care** and then on **Nurse-Client Interactions**.
• Select and view the video titled **0810: Monitoring/Patient Support**. (*Note:* Check the
virtual clock to see whether enough time has elapsed. You can use the fast-forward feature to
advance the time by 2-minute intervals if the video is not yet available. Then click again on
Patient Care and **Nurse-Client Interactions** to refresh the screen.)

3. What does Dorothy Grant say that she should do to help keep the violence away?

4. What are her concerns at this moment?

• Click on **Chart** and then on **201**.
- Click on the **History and Physical** and **Nursing Admission** tabs and review the information given.

5. According to the textbook, battered women share many characteristics. Compare the following list of characteristics from your textbook with Dorothy Grant's situation (based on your review of the Nursing Admission and History and Physical). For each characteristic listed, write Yes or No to indicate whether or not it applies to Dorothy Grant. For all Yes answers, provide a rationale to explain how that characteristic applies to her. (*Hint:* You may want to watch the 0810 video again.)

Textbook Characteristics of Battered Women	If/How Each Characteristic Applies to Dorothy Grant
Financially dependent	
Few resources/support systems	
Blame themselves for what has taken place	
State they are not "good enough"	
Bonding occurs out of fear and helplessness	
Low self-esteem	
History of domestic violence in their family	
Fear societal rejection	
Strong nurturing, yielding personality	

Textbook Characteristics of Battered Women	If/How Each Characteristic Applies to Dorothy Grant
Tolerate control from others easily	
Attempts to avoid arousing anger in the abuser	
Deliberate/repeated physical or sexual assault	

 Review the information regarding battering on pages 111-112 in your textbook.

6. Dorothy Grant stays in the abusive relationship because she feels that she has

_____.

7. What is the time period of greatest danger for the battered woman?

Let's jump ahead in virtual time to review some records that are not available until later in the day.

 • Click on **Return to Nurses' Station**; then click on **Leave the Floor** and **Restart the Program** to return to the sign-in window.)
• Sign in to work at Pacific View Regional Hospital on the Obstetrics Floor for Period of Care 3.
• From the Patient List, select Dorothy Grant (Room 201).
• Click on **Go to Nurses' Station**.
• Click on **Chart** and then on **201** to view Dorothy Grant's chart.
• Click on the **Consultations** tab and review the Psychiatric Consult and Social Work Consult.

8. According to these consultations, Dorothy Grant has several options. What do the social worker and psychiatric health care provider suggest to her or assist her with?

9. Indicate whether each of the following statements is true or false.

a. _____ Battering often escalates or begins during pregnancy.

b. _____ Dorothy Grant's husband blames her for the pregnancy.

c. _____ Dorothy Grant stays in the relationship because she likes to be beaten and deliberately provokes the attacks on occasion.

Exercise 3

CD-ROM Activity

30 minutes

- Sign in to work at Pacific View Regional Hospital on the Obstetrics Floor for Period of Care 4. (*Note:* If you are already in the virtual hospital from a previous exercise, click on **Leave the Floor** and then **Restart the Program** to get to the sign-in window.)
- Click on **Kardex** and then on **201** to review Dorothy Grant's Kardex. (*Remember:* You are not able to visit patients or administer medications during Period of Care 4. You are able to review patients' records only.)

1. What action was initiated on Wednesday to protect Dorothy Grant from her husband?

2. What care plan diagnoses are appropriate for Dorothy Grant's current life situation?

3. Members of what other disciplines have been contacted or consulted and will ensure continuity of care for Dorothy Grant as it relates to her abuse?

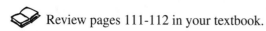 Review pages 111-112 in your textbook.

4. What is your responsibility, as a nurse, for reporting battering?

5. What are the reporting requirements of the state in which you practice?

6. What resources are available in your area for women who are experiencing battering?

LESSON 7

Nursing Management of Pain During Labor and Birth

 Reading Assignment: Nursing Management of Pain During Labor and Birth
(Chapter 7)

Patients: Kelly Brady, Obstetrics Floor, Room 203
Gabriela Valenzuela, Obstetrics Floor, Room 205
Laura Wilson, Obstetrics Floor, Room 206

Objectives:

- Assess and identify factors that influence pain perception.
- Describe selected nonpharmacologic and pharmacologic measures for pain management during labor and birth.

In this lesson you will compare and contrast the pain management strategies used with three patients during labor and birth.

Exercise 1

 CD-ROM Activity

30 minutes

- Sign in to work at Pacific View Regional Hospital on the Obstetrics Floor for Period of Care 1. (*Note:* If you are already in the virtual hospital from a previous exercise, click on **Leave the Floor** and then **Restart the Program** to get to the sign-in window.)
- From the Patient List, select Laura Wilson (Room 206).
- Click on **Get Report** and read the clinical report.

1. What is Laura Wilson's condition, according to the clinical report?

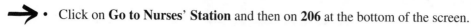

- Click on **Go to Nurses' Station** and then on **206** at the bottom of the screen.
- Inside the patient's room, read the Initial Observations.

2. What is your impression of Laura Wilson's condition?

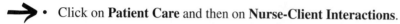

- Click on **Patient Care** and then on **Nurse-Client Interactions**.
- Select and view the video titled **0730: Patient Assessment**. (*Note:* Check the virtual clock to see whether enough time has elapsed. You can use the fast-forward feature to advance the time by 2-minute intervals if the video is not yet available. Then click again on **Patient Care** and **Nurse-Client Interactions** to refresh the screen.)

3. What is Laura Wilson's assessment of her current condition? How does this compare with the information you received from the clinical report and the Initial Observations summary?

- Click on **Chart** and then on **206** to view Laura Wilson's chart.
- Click on the **Nursing Admission** tab and review the information given.

4. List Laura Wilson's admission diagnoses. (*Hint:* See page 1 of the Nursing Admission form.)

5. What is your perception of Laura Wilson's behavior? What data have led you to this perception?

6. Think about the following questions and then discuss your ideas with your classmates: Do your personal values and beliefs contribute to your perception of Laura Wilson's behavior? If so, how? What nursing interventions might help to overcome your personal biases when dealing with Laura Wilson?

Exercise 2

 CD-ROM Activity

 30 minutes

 Review the sections on skin stimulation and breathing techniques on pages 159-162 in your textbook.

1. Effleurage is a variation of massage that stimulates _____

   nerve fibers that inhibit painful stimuli from traveling through

   _____ nerve fibers.

2. Different approaches to childbirth preparation use varying _____ techniques to help the woman maintain _____ through

   _____. _____ is the technique most associated with prepared childbirth. All patterns begin and end with a

   _____.

• Sign in to work at Pacific View Regional Hospital on the Obstetrics Floor for Period of Care 2. (*Note:* If you are already in the virtual hospital from a previous exercise, click on **Leave the Floor** and then **Restart the Program** to get to the sign-in window.)
• From the Patient List, select Gabriela Valenzuela (Room 205).
• Click on **Get Report** and read the clinical report.

 Review the section on systemic analgesia on pages 163-167 in your textbook.

3. Is Gabriela Valenzuela in labor at this time? Give a rationale for your answer.

 • Click on **Go to Nurses' Station** and then on **205** at the bottom of the screen.
• Click on **Patient Care** and then on **Nurse-Client Interactions**.
• Select and view the video titled **1140: Intervention—Bleeding, Comfort**. (*Note:* Check the virtual clock to see whether enough time has elapsed. You can use the fast-forward feature to advance the time by 2-minute intervals if the video is not yet available. Then click again on **Patient Care** and **Nurse-Client Interactions** to refresh the screen.)
• Click on **Chart** and then on **205** to view Gabriela Valenzuela's chart.
• Click on the **Nurse's Notes** tab and review the entry for 1140 on Wednesday.

4. How is Gabriela Valenzuela tolerating labor at this time?

5. What pain interventions is the nurse implementing at this time?

6. What is the action of fentanyl? (*Hint:* Review the Medication Guide on fentanyl on page 163 in your textbook.)

Let's begin the process of preparing and administering Gabriela Valenzuela's fentanyl dose.

 • Click on **Return to Room 205** and then on **Medication Room**.
• Click on **MAR** and then on **205**.
• Review the PRN medication administration record for Wednesday.

7. What is the ordered dose of fentanyl?

 • Click on **Return to Medication Room**.
- Click on **Automated System** and then on **Login**.
- In step 1, select **Gabriela Valenzuela, 205**. In step 2, select **Automated System Drawer (A-F)**.
- Click **Open Drawer**.
- Select **Fentanyl citrate**; then click **Put Medication on Tray**.
- Click on **Close Drawer**.
- Click on **View Medication Room** and then on **Preparation**.
- Click on **Prepare** and follow the Preparation Wizard prompts.
- Click on **Return to Medication Room** and then on **205** to go to the patient's room.

8. What additional assessments must be completed before you give Gabriela Valenzuela's medication?

9. Why is it important to check Gabriela Valenzuela's respirations before giving the dose of fentanyl?

10. What safety precautions should be in effect for Gabriela Valenzuela after she receives this dose of fentanyl?

• Click on **Patient Care** and then on **Medication Administration**.

• Click on **Review Your Medications** and then on the **Prepared** tab to verify the accuracy of your preparation.

• Click **Return to Room 205**.

• Click on the arrow next to Select and choose **Administer** from the drop-down menu.

• Follow the Administration Wizard prompts to administer Gabriela Valenzuela's fentanyl dose. Click **Yes** when asked whether to document this administration in the MAR.

• Click on **Patient Care** and then on **Nurse-Client Interactions**.

• Select and view the video titled **1155: Evaluation—Comfort Measures**. (*Note:* Check the virtual clock to see whether enough time has elapsed. You can use the fast-forward feature to advance the time by 2-minute intervals if the video is not yet available. Then click again on **Patient Care** and **Nurse-Client Interactions** to refresh the screen.)

11. Based on this video interaction, how effective were the nursing interventions that you identified in question 5 above?

12. Gabriela Valenzuela is experiencing _____.

_____ is responsible for the dizziness, as well as

other side effects, including _____,

_____, and numbness around the

_____ and _____.

13. What interventions does the nurse suggest to deal with the above problem that Gabriela Valenzuela is experiencing? List other interventions as described in your textbook.

At the end of the 1155 video, Gabriela Valenzuela states that she "doesn't want any needles" in her back. Learn more about this procedure by reading the Epidural Analgesia/Anesthesia section on pages 165-167 in your textbook.

14. What could you tell Gabriela Valenzuela to help her make an informed decision about anesthesia for labor? In the table below, list advantages and disadvantages of epidural anesthesia.

Advantages	Disadvantages

Let's see how you did preparing and administering the patient's medication.

- Click on **Leave the Floor** then **Look at Your Preceptor's Evaluation**.
- Click on **Medication Scorecard** and review the evaluation. How did you do?

Exercise 3

 CD-ROM Activity

 30 minutes

 Read the General Anesthesia section on pages 167-171 in your textbook.

- Sign in to work at Pacific View Regional Hospital on the Obstetrics Floor for Period of Care 4. (*Note:* If you are already in the virtual hospital from a previous exercise, click on **Leave the Floor** and then **Restart the Program** to get to the sign-in window.)
- Click on **Chart** and then on **203** to view Kelly Brady's chart. (*Remember:* You are not able to visit patients or administer medications during Period of Care 4. You are able to review patients' records only.)
- Click on the **Nurse's Notes** tab and review the entry for 1730 on Wednesday.

 1. Why does the anesthesiologist plan to use general anesthesia during Kelly Brady's cesarean section? (*Hint:* Read the Contraindications to Epidural Blocks section on page 166-167 in your textbook.)

2. Why is Kelly Brady upset about receiving general anesthesia for her surgery?

→ • Click on the **Physician's Orders** tab and review the entry for Wednesday at 1540.

3. What preoperative medications have been ordered for Kelly Brady?

→ • Click on **Return to Nurses' Station**.
- Click on the **Drug** icon in the lower left corner of your screen.
- Review the medications that you listed in the previous answer.

4. All of the medications listed below are given preoperatively to help prevent aspiration pneumonia. Using information from the Drug Guide and from the General Anesthesia section in your textbook, match each medication with the description of how it specifically works to prevent aspiration pneumonia.

Medication	Use in Preventing Pneumonia
_____ Sodium citrate/citric acid (Bicitra)	a. Decreases the production of gastric acid
_____ Metoclopramide (Reglan)	b. Prevents nausea and vomiting; accelerates gastric emptying
_____ Ranitidine (Zantac)	c. Neutralizes acidic stomach contents

5. How would you expect general anesthesia to affect Kelly Brady's baby? Why?

Nursing Care of Women with Complications During Labor and Birth

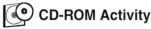 **Reading Assignment:** Nursing Care of Women with Complications During Labor and Birth (Chapter 8)

Patients: Dorothy Grant, Obstetrics Floor, Room 201
Stacey Crider, Obstetrics Floor, Room 202
Kelly Brady, Obstetrics Floor, Room 203
Gabriela Valenzuela, Obstetrics Floor, Room 205

Objectives:

- Assess and identify signs and symptoms present in the patient with preterm labor.
- Describe appropriate nursing care for the patient in preterm labor.
- Develop a birth plan to meet the needs of the preterm infant.

Exercise 1

 CD-ROM Activity

30 minutes

- Sign in to work at Pacific View Regional Hospital on the Obstetrics Floor for Period of Care 2. (*Note:* If you are already in the virtual hospital from a previous exercise, click on **Leave the Floor** and then **Restart the Program** to get to the sign-in window.)
- From the Patient List, select Dorothy Grant (Room 201) and Gabriela Valenzuela (Room 205).
- Click on **Go to Nurses' Station**.
- Click on **Chart** and then on **201** to view Dorothy Grant's chart.
- Click on the **History and Physical** tab and review the information given.

1. Using the information found in the History and Physical section, complete the table below for Dorothy Grant.

Patient	Weeks Gestation	Reason for Admission
Dorothy Grant		

- Click on **Chart** and then on **205** to view Gabriela Valenzuela's chart.
- Click on the **History and Physical** tab and review the information given.

2. Using the information found in the History and Physical section, complete the table below for Gabriela Valenzuela.

Patient	Weeks Gestation	Reason for Admission
Gabriela Valenzuela		

- Click on **Return to Nurses' Station** and then on **201** to enter Dorothy Grant's room.
- Click on **Patient Care** and then on **Pelvic** to perform a pelvic examination.

3. Complete the table below with the results of Dorothy Grant's initial cervical exam.

Patient	Time	Dilation	Effacement	Station
Dorothy Grant	0730			

- Click on **Nurses' Station** and then on **205** to enter Gabriela Valenzuela's room.
- Click on **Patient Care** and then on **Pelvic** to perform a pelvic examination.

4. Record the results of Gabriela Valenzuela's initial cervical examination in the table below.

Patient	Time	Dilation	Effacement	Station
Gabriela Valenzuela	0800			

Read the Preterm Labor section on pages 192-194 in your textbook.

5. What criteria are necessary to make a diagnosis of preterm labor?

6. As of Wednesday at 0800, would you consider both or either of these patients to be in preterm labor? Give a rationale for your answer.

Read the Tocolytic Therapy section on page 193 in your textbook to answer the following questions.

7. Match each medication below with the description of how it works as a tocolytic agent. Answers may be used more than once. (*Hint:* You may need to review the Drug Guide.)

_____ Magnesium sulfate

_____ Nifedipine (Procardia)

_____ Ritodrine (Yutopar)

_____ Terbutaline (Brethine)

_____ Indomethacin (Indocin)

a. Inhibits calcium from entering smooth muscle cells, thus relaxing uterine contractions

b. Relaxes uterine smooth muscle as a result of stimulation of beta 2 receptors on uterine smooth muscle

c. Exact mechanism unclear, but promotes relaxation of smooth muscles

d. Suppresses preterm labor by blocking the production of prostaglandins

Exercise 2

 CD-ROM Activity

30 minutes

- Sign in to work at Pacific View Regional Hospital on the Obstetrics Floor for Period of Care 1. (*Note:* If you are already in the virtual hospital from a previous exercise, click on **Leave the Floor** and then **Restart the Program** to get to the sign-in window.)
- From the Patient List, select Stacey Crider (Room 202).
- Click on **Get Report** and read the clinical report.

Stacey Crider was admitted yesterday in preterm labor and put on magnesium sulfate. Her other admission diagnoses were bacterial vaginosis and gestational diabetes with poorly controlled blood glucose levels.

1. What is Stacey Crider's current status in regard to preterm labor?

 - Click on **Go to Nurses' Station**.
- Click on **Chart** and then on **202** to view Stacey Crider's chart.
- Click on the **Physician's Orders** tab and review the orders for Wednesday at 0715.

2. Which of these orders relates specifically to Stacey Crider's diagnosis of preterm labor?

 - Now review the **Physician's Orders** for Wednesday at 0730.

3. What medication changes were ordered?

Read about terbutaline and nifedipine in the Tocolytic Therapy for Preterm Labor Medication Guide on page 193 in your textbook.

4. Why do you think Stacey Crider's physician changed his orders so quickly?

➤ • Click on **Return to Nurses' Station** and then on **202** to enter Stacy Crider's room.
  • Click on **Take Vital Signs**.

5. What are Stacey Crider's current vital signs? (*Note:* Answers will vary depending on the exact time you take the vital signs.)

Temperature:

Heart rate:

Respirations:

Blood pressure:

6. Which of the above parameters provides the most crucial information before giving Stacey Crider the nifedipine dose? Why? (*Hint:* Read about nifedipine on page 193 in your textbook.)

📖 Like Dorothy Grant and Kelly Brady, Stacey Crider is also receiving betamethasone. Read the Speeding Fetal Lung Maturity section in your textbook on pages 193-194.

7. Why are all three of these patients receiving antenatal glucocorticoid therapy?

➤ • Click on **MAR** and then on **202** to review Stacey Crider's MAR.

8. What is Stacey Crider's prescribed betamethasone dosage?

➤ • Click on **Return to Room 202** and then on **Medication Room**.
  • Click on **Unit Dosage** and then on drawer **202**.
  • Click on **Betamethasone**; then click **Put Medication on Tray**.
  • Click on **Close Drawer**.
  • Click on **View Medication Room** and then on Preparation.
  • Click on **Prepare** and follow the Preparation Wizard prompts.
  • Click on **Return to Medication Room**.

- Click on **202** to return to Stacey Crider's room.
- Click on **Check Armband** and then on **Check Allergies**.
- Click on **Patient Care**; then click **Medication Administration**.
- Click the arrow next to Select and choose **Administer**.
- Follow the Administration Wizard prompts. Check **Yes** to document the injection in the MAR.
- Click on **Leave the Floor**.
- Select **Look at Your Preceptor's Evaluation** and then click on **Medication Scorecard**. How did you do?

Exercise 3

 CD-ROM Activity

 15 minutes

- Sign in to work at Pacific View Regional Hospital on the Obstetrics Floor for Period of Care 4. (*Note:* If you are already in the virtual hospital from a previous exercise, click on **Leave the Floor** and then **Restart the Program** to get to the sign-in window.)
- Click on **Chart** and then on **201** to view Dorothy Grant's chart.
- Click on the **Nurse's Notes** tab and review the note for Wednesday 1815.

1. What is the result of Dorothy Grant's cervical exam at this time?

 • Review the **Nurse's Notes** for Wednesday 1840. It states that Dorothy Grant is being prepped for delivery.

2. If you were the nurse caring for Dorothy Grant during delivery, what special preparations would you make to care for the baby immediately after birth?

→ • Click on **Return to Nurses' Station**.
  • Click on **Chart** and then on **205** to view Gabriela Valenzuela's chart.
  • Click on the **Physician's Notes** tab and review the note for Wednesday 0800.

  3. What is the anticipated outcome of Gabriela Valenzuela's labor, according to this note?

→ • Review the **Physician's Notes** for Wednesday 1415 and 1455.

  4. What preparations have been made during the day for the birth of Gabriela Valenzuela's baby?

→ • Click on **Return to Nurses' Station**.
  • Click on **Chart** and then on **203** to view Kelly Brady's chart.
  • Click on the **Physician's Notes** tab and review the note for Wednesday 1530.

Read the Cesarean Birth section on pages 180-194 in your textbook.

  5. Why does Kelly Brady's physician now recommend immediate delivery?

  6. What general risks related to cesarean section does Kelly Brady's physician discuss with her?

7. Because of Kelly Brady's early gestational age (26 weeks), her physician anticipates a classical uterine incision. How will this type of incision affect Kelly Brady's birth options in future pregnancies?

 • Click on the **Physician's Orders** tab and review the orders for Wednesday 1540.

8. List the orders to be carried out before Kelly Brady's surgery. State the purpose of each order.

Order	Purpose

9. Can you think of other common preoperative procedures? List them below. (*Hint:* Refer to a basic medical-surgical textbook for ideas if you need help!)

LESSON 9

The Family After Birth

 Reading Assignment: The Family After Birth (Chapter 9)

Patient: Maggie Gardner, Obstetrics Floor, Room 204

Objectives:

- Identify the various types of loss as they relate to pregnancy.
- Describe the grieving process.
- Identify various methods of coping exhibited by patients who have experienced the loss of a newborn.

Exercise 1

 Writing Activity

15 minutes

 Review pages 212-213 in your textbook.

1. Parents may grieve not only for the death of a newborn, but also for a child born with a

    _____.

2. At what other times might couples grieve a pregnancy-related loss?

3. Women have many questions when they experience a pregnancy-related loss. What is the primary question asked?

4. _____ All women and men who undergo a loss receive the support that they need. (True or False)

Exercise 2

CD-ROM Activity

45 minutes

- Sign in to work at Pacific View Regional Hospital on the Obstetrics Floor for Period of Care 4. (*Note:* If you are already in the virtual hospital from a previous exercise, click on **Leave the Floor** and then **Restart the Program** to get to the sign-in window.)
- Click on **Chart** and then on **204** to review Maggie Gardner's chart. (*Remember:* You are not able to visit patients or administer medications during Period of Care 4. You are able to review patients' records only.)
- Click on the **History and Physical** tab and review this section.

  1. How many losses related to pregnancy has Maggie Gardner experienced?

- Click on the **Nursing Admission** tab and review the information given.

  2. Based on your review of the Nursing Admission, what is the first evidence that Maggie Gardner's previous losses are affecting her current pregnancy and care? (*Hint:* Review the first five sections of the Nursing Admission.)

- Click on the **Consultations** tab and review the Pastoral Consult.

  3. To what does Maggie Gardner attribute her inability to have a child?

  4. List three therapeutic measures that the chaplain can use to assist Maggie Gardner with these feelings as part of her grieving process?

5. What did the chaplain accomplish during his time with Maggie Gardner?

Exercise 3

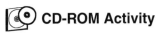 **CD-ROM Activity**

 30 minutes

Review pages 212-213 in your textbook.

1. List several common reactions to grieving.

2. What emotional responses typically emerge during intense grief?

3. Grieving is often chronic for parents of an infant with a birth defect. Why?

• Sign in to work at Pacific View Regional Hospital on the Obstetrics Floor for Period of Care 4. (*Note:* If you are already in the virtual hospital from a previous exercise, click on **Leave the Floor** and then **Restart the Program** to get to the sign-in window.)

• Click on **Chart** and then on **204**. (*Remember:* You are not able to visit patients or administer medications during Period of Care 4. You are able to review patients' records only.)

• Click on and review the **History and Physical** tab.

• Also click on **Consultations** and review the Pastoral Consult.

4. Compare Maggie Gardner's History and Physical with what typically happens during the reorganization phase. What correlation do you see?

5. Culture and religion play very important roles in how individuals handle a loss. How has Maggie Gardner handled her losses? (*Hint:* See "Effects of Illness on Spirituality" in the Pastoral Care Spiritual Assessment.)

10

Sexually Transmitted and Other Infections

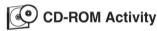 **Reading Assignment:** The Nurse's Role in Women's Health Care (Chapter 11, pages 254-258)

Patients: Stacey Crider, Obstetrics Floor, Room 202
Gabriela Valenzuela, Obstetrics Floor, Room 205
Laura Wilson, Obstetrics Floor, Room 206

Objectives:

- Assess and plan care for a pregnant woman with bacterial vaginosis.
- Explain the importance of prophylactic Group B streptococcus treatment.
- Identify risk factors for acquiring HIV infection.
- Prioritize information to be included in patient teaching related to HIV infection.

In this lesson, you will assess and evaluate the care provided to three hospitalized pregnant women, each of whom has a sexually transmitted infection (STI) or other vaginal infection.

Exercise 1

 CD-ROM Activity

20 minutes

- Sign in to work at Pacific View Regional Hospital on the Obstetrics Floor for Period of Care 1. (*Note:* If you are already in the virtual hospital from a previous exercise, click on **Leave the Floor** and then **Restart the Program** to get to the sign-in window.)
- From the Patient List, select Stacey Crider (Room 202).
- Click on **Go to Nurses' Station**.
- Click on **Chart** and then on **202** to view Stacey Crider's chart.
- Click on the **History and Physical** tab and review the information given.

115

1. Describe Stacey Crider's vaginal discharge on admission. How does it compare with the description of bacterial vaginosis found in Table 11-1 in your textbook?

	Stacey Crider's Discharge	Textbook Description
Appearance		
Amount		
Odor		

2. How is bacterial vaginosis diagnosed?

3. Which medication is recommended for treating bacterial vaginosis during pregnancy?

→ • Click on the **Physician's Orders** tab and review the admitting physician's orders on Tuesday at 0630.

4. What are Stacey Crider's admission diagnoses?

5. Explain how Stacey Crider's admission diagnoses are likely related.

6. Which medication did Stacey Crider's physician order to treat her bacterial vaginosis?

7. Assume that Stacey Crider is discharged home on day 4 of the prescribed treatment with this medication. What specific information about this drug should she be taught?

Exercise 2

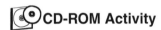 **CD-ROM Activity**

 20 minutes

- Sign in to work at Pacific View Regional Hospital on the Obstetrics Floor for Period of Care 1. (*Note:* If you are already in the virtual hospital from a previous exercise, click on **Leave the Floor** and then **Restart the Program** to get to the sign-in window.)
- From the Patient List, select Gabriela Valenzuela (Room 205).
- Click on **Go to Nurses' Station**.
- Click on **Chart** and then on **205** to view Gabriela Valenzuela's chart.
- Click on the **History and Physical** tab and review the plan outlined at the end of this document.

1. What is the medical plan of care for Gabriela Valenzuela?

2. Is Gabriela Valenzuela known to be positive for Group B streptococcus (GBS)?

Read about Group B streptococcus on pages 106 in your textbook.

3. List the risk factors for neonatal GBS infection.

4. Since pregnant women with GBS in the vagina are almost always asymptomatic, why does Gabriela Valenzuela need to be treated for this organism?

 • Click on the **Physician's Orders** tab and review the admission orders for Tuesday at 2100.

5. What medication/dosage/frequency will Gabriela Valenzuela receive for Group B strep prophylaxis?

6. How does this order compare with the treatment regimen recommended in your textbook?

Exercise 3

 CD-ROM Activity

 45 minutes

• Sign in to work at Pacific View Regional Hospital on the Obstetrics Floor for Period of Care 1. (*Note:* If you are already in the virtual hospital from a previous exercise, click on **Leave the Floor** and then **Restart the Program** to get to the sign-in window.)
• From the Patient List, select Laura Wilson (Room 206).
• Click on **Go to Nurses' Station**.
• Click on **Chart** and then on **206** to view Laura Wilson's chart.
• Click on the **Nursing Admission** tab and review the information given.

1. What risk factors for acquiring an STI are identified on Laura Wilson's Nursing Admission form?

2. List specific risk factors for acquiring HIV infection. (*Hint:* See page 106 in your textbook.) Underline the risk factors that are present in Laura Wilson's history.?

3. What did the admitting nurse document about Laura Wilson's knowledge and acceptance of her HIV diagnosis?

→ • Click on **Return to Nurses' Station**.
  • Click on **Patient Care** and then on **Nurse-Client Interactions**.
  • Select and view the video titled **0800: Teaching—HIV in Pregnancy**. (*Note:* Check the virtual clock to see whether enough time has elapsed. You can use the fast-forward feature to advance the time by 2-minute intervals if the video is not yet available. Then click again on **Patient Care** and **Nurse-Client Interactions** to refresh the screen.)

4. Does Laura Wilson appear to be fully aware of the implications of her HIV infection? State the rationale for your answer.

5. What coping mechanism is Laura Wilson exhibiting in the video clip?

→ • Click on **Chart** and then on **206** to view Laura Wilson's chart.
 • Click on the **Nursing Admission** tab and review the information given.

6. Laura Wilson needs education on all of the following topics. Which would you choose to teach her about at this time?
   a. Safer sex
   b. Medication side effects and importance of compliance
   c. Need for medical follow-up and medication for the baby
   d. Impact of HIV on birth plans

7. Give the rationale for your answer to the previous question.

Common Reproductive Concerns, Infertility, and Contraception

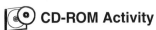 **Reading Assignment:** Human Reproductive Anatomy and Physiology (Chapter 2)
The Nurse's Role in Women's Health Care (Chapter 11)

Patients: Dororthy Grant, Obstetrics Floor, Room 201
Stacey Crider, Obstetrics Floor, Room 202
Kelly Brady, Obstetrics Floor, Room 203
Maggie Gardner, Obstetrics Floor, Room 204
Gabriela Valenzuela, Obstetrics Floor, Room 205
Laura Wilson, Obstetrics Floor, Room 206

Objectives:

- Identify reproductive concerns that can occur.
- Differentiate among the various types of contraception available.
- Identify various methods of testing and treatment options that can be used for couples experiencing infertility concerns.

Exercise 1

 CD-ROM Activity

 15 minutes

Review pages 26-28 and 251-253 in your textbook.

1. What is a normal length for a menstrual cycle?

2. What are the criteria for a diagnosis of amenorrhea?

 • Sign in to work at Pacific View Regional Hospital on the Obstetrics Floor for Period of Care 1. (*Note:* If you are already in the virtual hospital from a previous exercise, click on **Leave the Floor** and then **Restart the Program** to get to the sign-in window.)
 • From the Patient List, select Stacey Crider (Room 202).
 • Click on **Go to Nurses' Station**.
 • Click on **Chart** and then on **202** to view Stacey Crider's chart.
 • Click on the **History and Physical** tab and review the GYN History.

3. Does Stacey Crider meet the textbook criteria for amenorrhea?

4. What is her history?

Exercise 2

 CD-ROM Activity

 30 minutes

 Review pages 259-267 in your textbook.

1. What is contraception?

2. Providing contraception does not necessarily mean preventing

_____.

• Sign in to work at Pacific View Regional Hospital on the Obstetrics Floor for Period of Care 1. (*Note:* If you are already in the virtual hospital from a previous exercise, click on **Leave the Floor** and then **Restart the Program** to get to the sign-in window.)

• From the Patient List, select all six patients (although you will simply be reviewing the charts.)

• Click on **Go to Nurses' Station**.

• Click on **Chart** and then on **201** to view Dorothy Grant's chart.

• Click on the **History and Physical** tab and review the information on contraception.

• Repeat the previous three steps with each of the other five patients on the floor.

3. In the table below, list the birth control method each patient was using before this pregnancy.

Dorothy Grant

Stacey Crider

Kelly Brady

Maggie Gardner

Gabriela Valenzuela

Laura Wilson

4. Only _____ methods of contraception provide protection against STIs.

5. _____ is the only 100% effective method of preventing pregnancy and STIs.

6. Gabriela Gabriela is a devout Catholic. Which method of birth control would be appropriate for the nurse to discuss with her?

7. On what does this method rely?

Review pages 261-264 in your textbook.

8. Kelly Brady wants to use oral contraceptives to prevent pregnancy while she is also breast-feeding. Which type of oral contraception is appropriate for her to use? Why?

9. Laura Wilson is HIV-positive. What is the most appropriate form of birth control for her? Why?

Exercise 3

 CD-ROM Activity

 45 minutes

 Review the information on pages 267-272 in your textbook.

1. A fertile couple has a _____% chance of conception in each ovulatory cycle.

2. What are some psychologic reactions to infertility?

3. List four factors that affect female fertility.

4. List four factors that affect male fertility.

 • Sign in to work at Pacific View Regional Hospital on the Obstetrics Floor for Period of Care 1. (*Note:* If you are already in the virtual hospital from a previous exercise, click on **Leave the Floor** and then **Restart the Program** to get to the sign-in window.)
   • From the Patient List, select Maggie Gardner (Room 204).
   • Click on **Go to Nurses' Station**.
   • Click on **Chart** and then on **204** to view Maggie Gardner's chart.
   • Click on the **History and Physical** tab and review the information given.

5. Maggie Gardner was married _____ years before conceiving the first time.

6. Based on the textbook reading, which of the following would Maggie Gardner have been diagnosed with if she had chosen to get treatment after a year of attempting to get pregnant?
   a. Primary infertility
   b. Secondary infertility

7. List four factors that influence fertility.

8. Which of the above factors are known concerns with Maggie Gardner?

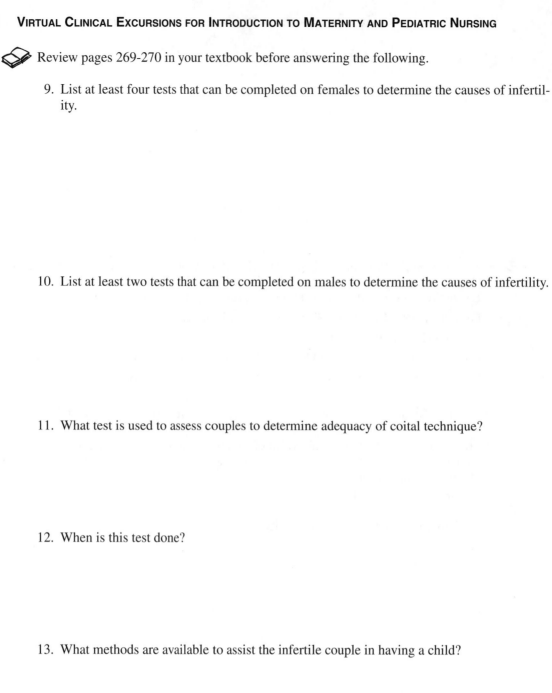 Review pages 269-270 in your textbook before answering the following.

9. List at least four tests that can be completed on females to determine the causes of infertility.

10. List at least two tests that can be completed on males to determine the causes of infertility.

11. What test is used to assess couples to determine adequacy of coital technique?

12. When is this test done?

13. What methods are available to assist the infertile couple in having a child?

14. What methods did Maggie Gardner and her husband use to assist in getting pregnant? (*Hint:* Review the OB history in her History and Physical.)

LESSON 12

Medication Administration

Patients: Dororthy Grant, Obstetrics Floor, Room 201
Stacey Crider, Obstetrics Floor, Room 202
Maggie Gardner, Obstetrics Floor, Room 204
Laura Wilson, Obstetrics Floor, Room 206

Objective:

- Correctly administer selected medications to obstetric patients observing the five rights.

Exercise 1

 CD-ROM Activity

 30 minutes

- Sign in to work at Pacific View Regional Hospital on the Obstetrics Floor for Period of Care 2. (*Note:* If you are already in the virtual hospital from a previous exercise, click on **Leave the Floor** and then **Restart the Program** to get to the sign-in window.)
- From the Patient List, select Dorothy Grant (Room 201).

Dorothy Grant was admitted at 30 weeks gestation for observation following blunt abdominal trauma (she was kicked in the abdomen by her husband). Dorothy Grant is bleeding vaginally and may have sustained a placental abruption. Your assignment is to give Rho(D) immune globulin to Dorothy Grant. Read about Rho(D) immune globulin on page 96 in your textbook and in the Drug Guide on your CD-ROM.

1. Rho(D) immune globulin is a solution of _____ given after delivery of an

   Rh-_____ fetus to an Rh-_____ mother to prevent the maternal Rh immune response.

2. All of the following are scenarios in which Rho(D) immune globulin might be administered. Which of these scenarios applies to Dorothy Grant?
   a. Administered within 72 hours of giving birth to an Rh-positive infant
   b. Given prophylactically at 28 weeks gestation
   c. Administered following an incident or exposure risk that occurs after 28 weeks gestation
   d. Given during first trimester pregnancy following miscarriage, elective abortion, or ectopic pregnancy

127

3. List the information about Dorothy Grant that must be determined before giving her Rho(D) immune globulin.

→ • Click on **Go to Nurses' Station**.
   • Click on **Chart** and then on **201** to view Dorothy Grant's chart.
   • Click on the **Physician's Orders** tab and review the orders for Wednesday 0730.

4. Write the Physician's Order for Rho(D) immune globulin.

→ • Click on the **Drug** icon in the lower left corner of your screen. Find the entry for Rho(D) immune globulin and compare the Physician's Order for Dorothy Grant with the dosage and route specified in the Drug Guide.

5. According to the Drug Guide, does the Physician's Order use the correct dosage and route?

→ • Click on the **Laboratory Reports** tab and review test results for 0245 Wednesday.

6. Dorothy Grant's blood type is _____.

7. What additional information do you need? Why? Is that information available?

→ • Click on **Return to Nurses' Station** and then on **Medication Room**.
   • Click on Refrigerator and open the refrigerator door.
   • Click on **Put Medication on Tray** and then on Close Door.
   • Click on **View Medication Room** and then on Preparation.
   • Click on Prepare and follow the prompts to complete preparation of this medication.
   • Click on **Return to Medication Room** and then on 201 to enter the patient's room.
   • Click on **Check Armband**.
   • Click on **Patient Care** and then on **Medication Administration**.

You are almost ready to give Dorothy Grant's injection. However, before you do . . .

8. _____ Rho(D) immune globulin is often considered a blood product. (True or False)

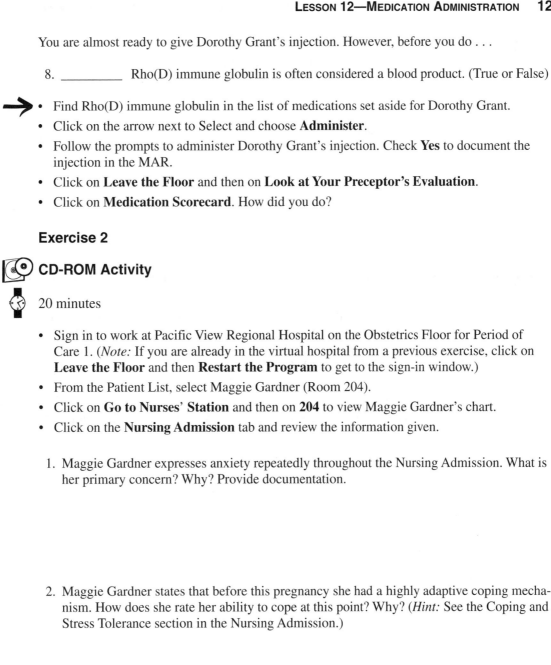

- Find Rho(D) immune globulin in the list of medications set aside for Dorothy Grant.
- Click on the arrow next to Select and choose **Administer**.
- Follow the prompts to administer Dorothy Grant's injection. Check **Yes** to document the injection in the MAR.
- Click on **Leave the Floor** and then on **Look at Your Preceptor's Evaluation**.
- Click on **Medication Scorecard**. How did you do?

Exercise 2

CD-ROM Activity

20 minutes

- Sign in to work at Pacific View Regional Hospital on the Obstetrics Floor for Period of Care 1. (*Note:* If you are already in the virtual hospital from a previous exercise, click on **Leave the Floor** and then **Restart the Program** to get to the sign-in window.)
- From the Patient List, select Maggie Gardner (Room 204).
- Click on **Go to Nurses' Station** and then on **204** to view Maggie Gardner's chart.
- Click on the **Nursing Admission** tab and review the information given.

1. Maggie Gardner expresses anxiety repeatedly throughout the Nursing Admission. What is her primary concern? Why? Provide documentation.

2. Maggie Gardner states that before this pregnancy she had a highly adaptive coping mechanism. How does she rate her ability to cope at this point? Why? (*Hint:* See the Coping and Stress Tolerance section in the Nursing Admission.)

- Click on the **Physician's Orders** tab and review the information given.

3. What medication has the physician ordered to help Maggie Gardner with her anxiety?

• Click on **Return to Nurses' Station**.

• Click on the **Drug** icon in the lower left corner of your screen.

• Use the search box or the scroll bar to find the medication you identified in the previous question.

4. What is the drug's mechanism of action?

 • Click on **Return to Nurses' Station** and then on **204** to enter Maggie Gardner's room.

• Click on **Patient Care** and then on **Nurse-Client Interactions**.

• Select and view the video titled **0745: Evaluation—Efficacy of Drugs**. (*Note:* Check the virtual clock to see whether enough time has elapsed. You can use the fast-forward feature to advance the time by 2-minute intervals if the video is not yet available. Then click again on **Patient Care** and **Nurse-Client Interactions** to refresh the screen.)

5. According to the nurse, how long will it take for Maggie Gardner to see therapeutic effects of the drug? How does this correlate with what you learned in the Teaching section of the Drug Guide?

Exercise 3

 CD-ROM Activity

 30 minutes

• Sign in to work at Pacific View Regional Hospital on the Obstetrics Floor for Period of Care 1. (*Note:* If you are already in the virtual hospital from a previous exercise, click on **Leave the Floor** and then **Restart the Program** to get to the sign-in window.)

• From the Patient List, select Stacey Crider (Room 202).

1. In this exercise, you will administer betamethasone to Stacey Crider, who was admitted to the hospital at 27 weeks gestation in preterm labor. Before preparing Stacey Crider's betamethasone, what do you need to do?

→ • Click on **Go to Nurses' Station**.
  • Click on **Chart** and then on **202** to view Stacey Crider's chart.
  • Click on the **Physician's Orders** tab and find the order for betamethasone.

  2. After verifying the Physician's Order, what is your next step?

→ • Click on **Return to Nurses' Station** and then on **Medication Room**.
  • Click on **Unit Dosage** and then on drawer **202**.
  • Select **Betamethasone**; then click on **Put Medication on Tray**.
  • Click on **Close Drawer**.
  • Click on **View Medication Room** and then on Preparation.
  • Click on Prepare and follow the prompts to complete preparation of Stacey Crider's betamethasone dose.
  • Click on **Return to Medication Room**.

  3. Now that the medication is prepared, what's your next step?

→ • Click on **202** to enter the patient's room.
  • Click on **Check Armband** and Check Allergies.
  • Click on **Patient Care** and then on **Medication Administration**.
  • Click **Select** for betamethasone and choose **Administer**.
  • Follow the prompts to administer Stacey Crider's betamethasone injection.

  4. What's the final step in the process?

→ • If you haven't already, indicate **Yes** to document the injection in the MAR.
  • Click on **Leave the Floor**.
  • Click on **Look at Your Preceptor's Evaluation**.
  • Click on **Medication Scorecard**. How did you do?

Exercise 4

 CD-ROM Activity

 30 minutes

- Sign in to work at Pacific View Regional Hospital on the Obstetrics Floor for Period of Care 1. (*Note:* If you are already in the virtual hospital from a previous exercise, click on **Leave the Floor** and then **Restart the Program** to get to the sign-in window.)
- From the Patient List, select Laura Wilson (Room 206).
- Click on **Go to Nurses' Station**.
- Click on **MAR** and then on **206** to view Laura Wilson's MAR.

1. Laura Wilson's medications for Wednesday include several different types of drugs. Which of the following is used to treat her HIV-positive status?
   a. Zidovudine 200 mg PO every 8 hours
   b. Prenatal multivitamin 1 tablet PO daily
   c. Lactated Ringer's 1000 mL IV continuous

 - Click on **Return to Nurses' Station**.
- Click on the **Drug** icon in the lower left corner of the screen.
- Use the search box or scroll bar to find the medication you identified in the previous question.

2. What is the drug's mechanism of action?

3. What is the drug's therapeutic effect?

4. Does this medication cross the placenta? Is it distributed in breast milk?

5. What symptoms/side effects of this medication need to be reported to the physician?

6. How should this medication be taken?

7. Your final assignment is to give Laura Wilson the medication that is due at 0800. During these lessons, we have provided you with detailed instructions on how to give medications. Now it is time for you to fly solo. Don't forget the five rights of medication administration . . . and have fun! Document below how you did.

Note: If you'd like to get more practice, there are other medications that can be given at the beginning of the first three periods of care. Below is a list of patients, medications, and routes of administration that can be used for more practice in Periods of Care 1, 2, and 3. As you practice, be sure to select the correct patient when you sign in. That way, you can get a Medication Score-card for evaluation after you prepare and administer a medication. (*Remember:* If you need help at any time, refer to pages 19-22, 26-30, and 37-41 in the **Getting Started** section of this workbook.)

PERIOD OF CARE 1

Dorothy Grant (Room 201)

- Betamethasone 12 mg IM
- Prenatal multivitamin PO

Stacey Crider (Room 202)

- Prenatal multivitamin PO
- Metronidazole 500 mg PO
- Betamethasone 12 mg IM
- Insulin lispro Sub-Q
- Nifedipine 20 mg PO

Kelly Brady (Room 203)

- Prenatal multivitamin PO
- Ferrous sulfate PO
- Labetalol hydrochloride 400 mg PO
- Nifedipine 10 mg PO

Maggie Gardner (Room 204)

- Prenatal multivitamin PO
- Buspirone hydrochloride 5 mg PO

Gabriela Valenzuela (Room 205)

- Ampicillin 2 grams IV
- Betamethasone 12 mg IM
- Prenatal multivitamin PO

Laura Wilson (Room 206)

- Zidovudine 200 mg PO
- Prenatal multivitamin PO

PERIOD OF CARE 2

Dorothy Grant (Room 201)

- Rho(D) immune globulin IM

Stacey Crider (Room 202)

- Insulin lispro Sub-Q

Kelly Brady (Room 203)

- Betamethasone 12 mg IM

Maggie Gardner (Room 204)

- Prednisone 40 mg PO
- Aspirin 81 mg PO

PERIOD OF CARE 3

Maggie Gardner (Room 204)

- Buspirone 5 mg PO

LESSON 13

Caring for an Infant with Bronchiolitis

∽ **Reading Assignment:** An Overview of Growth, Development, and Nutrition
(Chapter 15, pages 345-379)

The Infant (Chapter 16, pages 380-398)

Health Care Adaptations for the Child and Family (Chapter 22, pages 485, 486-491, 506-507, and 512-513)

The Child with a Respiratory or Cardiovascular Disorder (Chapter 25, pages 571-573 and 577-578)

The Child with a Communicable Disease (Chapter 31, pages 717-718)

Patient: Carrie Richards, Pediatrics Floor, Room 303

Objectives:

- Discuss the pathophysiology of bronchiolitis.
- Explain the role of respiratory syncytial virus (RSV) in bronchiolitis.
- Relate the effect of an infant's level of growth and development on bronchiolitis.
- Complete a respiratory assessment on an infant and discuss nursing care issues.
- Determine nursing interventions for an infant with bronchiolitis.

In this lesson you will learn and reinforce concepts related to a common respiratory illness in infants. You will apply principles of growth and development in making nursing care decisions. You will be expected to recall/review basic oral and written communication skills, teaching skills, and family-centered care. Your patient is Carrie Richards, a 3.5-month-old who has been admitted to the Pediatric Unit from the Emergency Department. Carrie's medical diagnosis is bronchiolitis. Her mother is with her.

Exercise 1

 Writing Activity

 15 minutes

1. Explain the pathophysiology of bronchiolitis.

2. What is the relationship between respiratory syncytial virus and bronchiolitis?

3. Discuss infant growth and development as it relates to respiratory tract function.

Exercise 2

 CD-ROM Activity

 30 minutes

- Sign in to work at Pacific View Regional Hospital on the Pediatrics Floor for Period of Care 1. (*Note:* If you are already in the virtual hospital from a previous exercise, click on **Leave the Floor** and then **Restart the Program** to get to the sign-in window.)
- From the Patient List, select Carrie Richards (Room 303).
- Click on **Go to Nurses' Station**.
- Click on **Chart** and then on **303**.
- Click on the **Emergency Department** tab and review the record.
- Click on and review the **Physician's Orders**, **History and Physical**, and **Nursing Admission**.

1. As you review these records, list the data that are consistent with bronchiolitis.

2. What do these observations indicate as far as Carrie Richards' health status is concerned? Do you think Carrie is mildly or severely ill? Explain.

→ • Click on the **Physician's Orders** and find the medications ordered for Carrie Richards.
- Click on **Return to Nurses' Station**.
- Review data on Carrie's ordered medications by clicking on the **Drug** icon in the lower left corner of your screen. (*Hint:* You may also refer to a nursing drug handbook if you need more information.)

3. What are the rationales for the orders for IV fluid, medications, pulse oximetry, and lab work?

4. Nasal washing was performed on Carrie Richards while she was in the ED. If you were assisting with the nasal washing procedure, would you anticipate restraining her? If so, how? Would you have Carrie's mother help? What factors would you consider in deciding what to do? (*Hint:* Check Carrie's physical status and behavior while she was in the ED.)

5. Explain the type of isolation being used for Carrie Richards. (*Hint:* To find this, check the Physician's Orders in her chart.)

6. What other infection-control precautions, aside from isolation, need to be implemented?

7. What is a nosocomial infection, and why must care be taken to prevent Carrie Richards from developing one?

- Click on **Return to Nurses' Station** and then on **303** at the bottom of the screen.
- Click on **Patient Care** and then on **Nurse-Client Interactions**.
- Select and view the video titled **0730: Patient Assessment**. (*Note:* Check the virtual clock to see whether enough time has elapsed. You can use the fast-forward feature to advance the time by 2-minute intervals if the video is not yet available. Then click again on **Patient Care** and **Nurse-Client Interactions** to refresh the screen.)

8. In this video, what are the nurse and Carrie Richards' mother doing right? What are they doing wrong?

Exercise 3

 CD-ROM Activity

 45 minutes

- Sign in to work at Pacific View Regional Hospital on the Pediatrics Floor for Period of Care 1. (*Note:* If you are already in the virtual hospital from a previous exercise, click on **Leave the Floor** and then **Restart the Program** to get to the sign-in window.)
- From the Patient List, select Carrie Richards (Room 303).
- Click on **Go to Nurses' Station**.
- Click on **303** to go to Carrie Richards' room.
- Inside the room, click on **Check Armband** and then on **Take Vital Signs**. Note Carrie Richards' vital signs for documentation.
- Next, click on **Patient Care** and perform a head-to-toe assessment by clicking on the various body areas and subcategories.

1. Based on your assessment, list any observations that reflect the status of Carrie Richards' oxygenation.

2. When taking Carrie Richards' temperature, which method is the most appropriate to use?
   a. Axillary
   b. Oral
   c. Rectal
   d. Tympanic

3. What is the proper position to hold the pinna of the ear when using a tympanic thermometer on Carrie Richards?
   a. Down and back
   b. Up and back
   c. Straight back

4. What are Carrie's vital signs? Are they within normal range for her age?

5. Carrie is of African-American descent. What is the best way to assess color in a dark-skinned person?

→ • Click on **EPR** and then on **Login**.
   • Specify **303** in the Patient box.
   • Begin charting the finding from your assessment of Carrie Richards by selecting **Vital Signs** in the Category box. Use the blue backward and forward arrows as needed to document these data in the appropriate time column.
   • Continue to chart your observations in the Respiratory and Cardiovascular categories.

6. If you missed anything, go back to Carrie Richards' room and reassess her. Because the EPR format is generic, you may not have data for all areas listed. Even so, you do need to make sure you are recognizing significant assessment data. Review data trends since admission. Why is continued monitoring necessary?

→ • Click **Exit EPR** to return to Carrie Richards' room.
   • Based on your previous findings and your answer to question 6, perform a focused assessment of Carrie Richards.
   • Click on **Leave the Floor**.
   • Click on **Look at Your Preceptor's Evaluation**s.
   • Click on and review the **Examination Report**.

7. How did you do with your focused assessment? Do you note any gaps? Were you efficient and systemic? Is there any need for improvement in your performance? If so, in what areas?

- Click on **Return to Evaluations**.
- Click on **Return to Menu** and **Restart the Program**.
- Sign in to work at Pacific View Regional Hospital on the Pediatric Floor for Period of Care 1.
- From the Patient List, select Carrie Richards (Room 303).
- Click on **Go to Nurses' Station**.
- Click on **EPR** and then on **Login**.
- Select Carrie Richard' EPR (**303**) and document your latest assessment findings.

8. Is Carrie Richards' condition improving or deteriorating?

9. Consider the possibility of Carrie's condition deteriorating. What changes might you anticipate that would indicate worsening of her health status?

10. How is Carrie Richards receiving oxygen?

11. Sometimes oxygen is delivered via a mist tent. What are the nursing responsibilities for care of an infant in a mist tent? Are there any advantages to using a mist tent rather than a nasal cannula?

12. How is Carrie Richards' O_2 status being monitored? What should the nurse be looking for?

13. Documentation is important. What information is necessary for documenting observations associated with Carrie Richards' O_2 saturation levels?

14. Oxygenation assessment is ongoing. In older children and adults, the nurse can easily assess respiratory status in response to play or other activity. How can this ongoing assessment be carried out in an infant?

15. Develop a list of the major nursing interventions for Carrie Richards.

Congratulations! You have just completed a comprehensive study of bronchiolitis in an infant. You have considered nursing care for this respiratory illness. Proceed to the next lesson to learn about other nursing care challenges and how to respond.

Nursing Care Issues Associated with Bronchiolitis

⟨∞ **Reading Assignment:** An Overview of Growth, Development, and Nutrition
(Chapter 15, pages 345-379)

The Infant (Chapter 16, pages 380-398)

Health Care Adaptations for the Child and Family (Chapter 22, pages 496-506 and 503-509)

The Child with a Gastrointestinal Condition (Chapter 27, pages 646-649)

The Child with a Communicable Disease (Chapter 31, pages 721-722)

Patient: Carrie Richards, Pediatrics Floor, Room 303

Objectives:

- Discuss the reasons why infants are at risk for hydration problems.
- Explain the risk for dehydration in infants with respiratory problems.
- Discuss nursing care for managing hydration concerns, including IV therapy.
- Practice oral medication administration in infants.
- Identify and discuss teaching implications in the care of infants.
- Discuss discharge information for the parent(s) of a patient with bronchiolitis.

In this lesson you will explore hydration as an area of concern in infants with respiratory problems. You will also explore oral medication administration and practice it in the virtual hospital setting. You will consider the role of the nurse related to a variety of teaching areas: the illness, oral administration of medications, and growth and development. You will need to recall and use the principles of good communication and family teaching as you continue to work with Carrie Richards.

Exercise 1

 Writing Activity

30 minutes

1. What are several characteristics of infants that put them at greater risk for hydration problems?

2. List the areas that you would review in a hydration assessment.

3. What is the most reliable information you can use to assess an infant's hydration over time? Why?

4. When is the best time to weigh an infant? How would you do this?

5. Explain what is meant by oral rehydration therapy (ORT).

6. Discuss the nursing responsibilities associated with IV fluid administration in infants. (*Hint:* Remember that IV fluid is treated as a medication administration.)

7. What should the nurse be looking for when assessing an IV site?

8. What topics should be included in discharge instructions after hospitalization with bronchiolitis?

Exercise 2

 CD-ROM Activity

30 minutes

- Sign in to work at Pacific View Regional Hospital on the Pediatrics Floor for Period of Care 1. (*Note:* If you are already in the virtual hospital from a previous exercise, click on **Leave the Floor** and then **Restart the Program** to get to the sign-in window.)
- From the Patient List, select Carrie Richards (Room 303).
- Click on **Get Report** and then on **Go to Nurses' Station**.
- Click on **303** at the bottom of your screen.
- Click on **Patient Care** and complete a focused assessment of Carrie Richards. (*Remember:* A focused assessment is one that reflects the priority health concern as well as those concerns for which the patient is at risk.)
- Once your assessment is complete, click on **EPR** and then on **Login**.
- Specify Carrie Richards' room number (**303**) and choose categories as needed to record the data from your focused assessment. (*Hint:* If you need help entering data in the EPR, refer to pages 15-16 in the **Getting Started** section of this workbook.)
- When you have finished documenting your assessments, click on **Exit EPR**.
- Now, to see how you did, first click on **Leave the Floor**.
- From the Floor Menu, select **Look at Your Preceptor's Evaluation**s.
- Now click on **Examination Report** and review the feedback.

1. Reflect on your performance with this assessment. Did you assess respiratory status along with hydration parameters? Remember that each affects the other.

2. What important hydration assessment parameters can you use with Carrie Richards that would not be available with an older child?

Now let's jump ahead in virtual time to practice your focused assessment again.

 - Click on **Return to Evaluations**, **Return to Menu**, and then **Restart the Program**.
- Sign in to work on the Pediatrics Floor for Period of Care 2.
- From the Patient List, select Carrie Richards (Room 303).

- Click on **Go to Nurses' Station** and then on **303** at the bottom of the screen to enter Carrie Richards' room.
- Click **Patient Care** and complete a focused assessment. Then chart your findings on the appropriate flow sheets in the EPR.
- When you have finished documenting your assessments, click on **Exit EPR**.
- Now, see how you did. Click on **Leave the Floor**.
- From the Floor Menu, select **Look at Your Preceptor's Evaluation**s.
- Now click on **Examination Report** and review the feedback.

3. Reflect on how you are doing with your focused assessment. Consider completeness, comfort, efficiency, and skill. Are you feeling more confident about your thoroughness?

4. You know that infusion pumps are in very short supply. You also know that Carrie Richards, because of her age, needs a pump and will get the next available one. In the meantime, she has IV tubing with a burette. What is the rationale for use of this type of tubing?

5. What would you tell Carrie Richards' mother about adequate hydration? How will she know whether or not her baby is getting enough fluids?

6. Carrie Richards is receiving an IV infusion with potassium added. Explain what she is receiving. Discuss the nurse's responsibilities related to potassium administration to an infant.

7. What can Carrie Richards' mother do regarding management of the IV? What could you ask her to do while still maintaining safe care and fulfilling your legal responsibility?

Exercise 3

 CD-ROM Activity

 45 minutes

- Sign in to work at Pacific View Regional Hospital on the Pediatrics Floor for Period of Care 3. (*Note:* If you are already in the virtual hospital from a previous exercise, click on **Leave the Floor** and then **Restart the Program** to get to the sign-in window.)
- From the Patient List, select Carrie Richards (Room 303).
- Click on **Go to Nurses' Station**.
- Click on **303** to go to Carrie Richards' room.
- Click on **Take Vital Signs**.
- Click on **Clinical Alerts** and review the report.

1. Can Carrie Richards be given Tylenol? If so, for what reason?

2. What should you assess before you prepare the medication? (*Hint:* Consider the specific need for this medication, as well as the nursing responsibilities before administering any medication.)

➤ • Click on **MAR** and then on **303**. Find the order for this medication.

3. Is the ordered dose of this medication appropriate for Carrie Richards? Why or why not?

4. Assume that Carrie Richards had an order for an antibiotic that reads "40 mg/kg/day PO in divided doses every 8 hours." How much would you give for each dose?

5. What are the appropriate methods for administering oral medications to an infant?

• Click on **Return to Room 303**.
- Click on **Medication Room**.
- Click on **Unit Dosage** and then on drawer **303**.
- Click on **Acetaminophen** and then on **Put Medication on Tray**.
- Click on **Close Drawer**.
- Click on **View Medication Room**; then click **Preparation**.
- Click on **Prepare** and follow the Preparation Wizard's prompts.
- Click on **Return to Medication Room**.
- Click on **303** to return to Carrie Richards's room.
- Click on **Check Armband** and **Check Allergies**.
- Click on **Patient Care** and then on **Medication Administration**.
- Find **Acetaminophen** listed on the left side of your screen. Click on the down arrow next to Select and choose **Administer**.
- Follow the Administration Wizard's prompts to administer the medication. Indicate **Yes** to document administration in the MAR.
- Click on **Leave the Floor**.
- Click on **Look at Your Preceptor's Evaluation**.
- Click on **Medication Scorecard**. How did you do?

6. Did you get check marks indicating that you completed the medication administration procedure satisfactorily? What, if anything, did you forget? What, if anything, would you do differently?

You have just been walked through the medication preparation and administration procedure. Now try it on your own. You can practice preparing and giving Carrie Richards the same aceta-minophen dose you just completed, or you can check the MAR to see whether there are any other medications that you can administer to her.

• Click on **Leave the Floor** and then **Restart the Program**. Sign in again to work with Carrie Richards for Period of Care 3 and proceed from there.
- Remember to follow the five rights! After you have finished administering the medication, be sure to see how you did by checking your Medication Scorecard.
- Click on **Leave the Floor** and then on **Look at Your Preceptor's Evaluation**s.
- Click on **Medication Scorecard** and review your evaluation.

Now let's jump backward in virtual time to visit Carrie Richards earlier in the day.

 • First, click on **Return to Evaluations**, then on **Return to Menu**, and then on **Restart the Program**.
• Sign in to work with Carrie Richards again, this time for Period of Care 2.
• Click on **Go to Nurses' Station** and then on **303** to go to Carrie Richards's room.
• Click on **Patient Care** and then on **Nurse-Client Interactions**.
• Select and view the video titled **1115: Nutritional Assessment**. (*Note:* Check the virtual clock to see whether enough time has elapsed. You can use the fast-forward feature to advance the time by 2-minute intervals if the video is not yet available. Then click again on **Patient Care** and **Nurse-Client Interactions** to refresh the screen.)

7. Share your thoughts on the nurse's teaching. Consider the teaching-learning principles that are depicted.

8. Carrie Richards' mother needs to know how to give medication to her child at home. How will you determine whether she is skillful and comfortable enough giving her baby medication?

9. How would you respond to the following concern: "The nurse is supposed to give the medication, so how can the nurse allow a parent to administer medication?" (*Hint:* To answer this, you need to think through the nurse's legal responsibilities.)

10. The only vaccine Carrie Richards has received is for hepatitis B. What teaching does Carrie Richards' mother need with regard to immunizations?

11. What other kinds of information would you want from Carrie Richards' mother? (*Hint:* Explore other factors contributing to her behavior and decision making.)

12. Suppose that Carrie Richards' mother expresses concern about pain. She says that she avoids getting Carrie's shots because of this fear. You have shared this information, and the RN has requested an order for EMLA cream prior to any injections. What information does Carrie Richards' mother need in order to use EMLA cream?

Great job on completing this lesson! These exercises have helped you to think about pediatric situations in the hospital setting.

15

Caring for an Infant
Who Is Failing to Thrive

 Reading Assignment: An Overview of Growth, Development, and Nutrition
(Chapter 15, pages 370-372)
The Child with a Gastrointestinal Condition (Chapter 27,
pages 649-650)

Patient: Carrie Richards, Pediatrics Floor, Room 303

Objectives:

* Discuss normal nutritional needs for the infant.
* Define failure to thrive (FTT).
* Consider patterns of growth that may indicate FTT.
* Determine areas of assessment when FTT is suspected.
* Discuss relationship of parenting skills to FTT.
* Develop specific interventions for caring for an infant with FTT.

As you complete this lesson, you will explore the complexities of failure to thrive, including the factors of parent-infant interaction and parenting skills. You will also consider the role of the nurse in assessment, support, and teaching when providing care.

Exercise 1

 Writing Activity

30 minutes

1. Why is adequate nutrition especially important in infancy?

2. Describe appropriate nutritional intake for an infant at 3.5 months of age.

3. Compare and contrast organic and nonorganic failure to thrive. How are they similar, and how are they different?

4. The following is a list of assessment data, some physiologic and some psychosocial. Place an X next to each piece of data that should be assessed further when there is a concern about failure to thrive.

_____ a. Weight less than 3rd-5th percentile

_____ b. Sudden deceleration in growth or weight loss

_____ c. Delay in reaching milestones

_____ d. Decreased muscle mass

_____ e. Muscle hypotonia

_____ f. Wary of caregivers

_____ g. Unresponsive to cuddling

_____ h. Nonnurturing parenting behaviors

_____ i. Avoidance of eye contact or touch

_____ j. Intense watchfulness

_____ k. Sleep disturbance

_____ l. Lack of age-appropriate stranger anxiety

5. Are there other areas that need to be assessed? If so, list some of these areas.

6. What are the potential long-term effects of untreated failure to thrive?

7. Discuss the impact of failure to thrive on growth and development. Consider areas of development in addition to height and weight parameters.

8. Review child abuse on page 566 in your textbook. The term child abuse can refer to emotional abuse and neglect, physical abuse and neglect, and sexual abuse. Is there abuse in Carrie Richards' situation? Is there risk for abuse? Share your reasons for thinking the way you do.

9. What is the nurse's responsibility if there is a suspicion of abuse? (*Hint:* Discuss documentation and reporting.)

10. Discuss your own thoughts and any possible biases concerning child abuse and neglect.

 11. On page 650 in your textbook, find the statement that says "It is vital to support rather that reject the mother." Comment on your ability to do this.

Exercise 2

 CD-ROM Activity

 30 minutes

- Sign in to work at Pacific View Regional Hospital on the Pediatrics Floor for Period of Care 2. (*Note:* If you are already in the virtual hospital from a previous exercise, click on **Leave the Floor** and then **Restart the Program** to get to the sign-in window.)
- From the Patient List, select Carrie Richards (Room 303).
- Click on **Go to Nurses' Station**.
- Click on **Chart** and then on **303**.
- Click on **Nursing Admission**.

1. If you knew Carrie Richards' birth weight, how would you use this information for assessment? What is the rule of thumb for expected weight gain in an infant?

2. Discuss the potential role of an interdisciplinary team providing care for Carrie Richards. Who might be involved?

→ • Now click on **Consultations**.
  • Review the Dietary/Nutrition Consult.

3. Find Carrie Richards' birth weight and current weight. Based on this information, what concerns do you have about her rate of growth?

4. You considered the recommended diet for a 3.5-month-old in question 2 of Exercise 1 in this lesson. How does this compare with Carrie Richards' diet? Evaluate the adequacy of her diet and consider her mother's rationales for these choices. Is there anything else you want to know or assess?

5. Based on your review of the Dietary/Nutrition Consult, what do you think is the problem in regard to Carrie Richards' feedings? What additional dietary recommendations are planned for her?

6. As you talk with Carrie Richards' mother, you learn that income is a problem. When discussing feeding, what should you incorporate in your teaching?

7. How will you teach Carrie Richards' mother about formula preparation?

Exercise 3

  CD-ROM Activity

 30 minutes

- Sign in to work at Pacific View Regional Hospital on the Pediatrics Floor for Period of Care 1. (*Note:* If you are already in the virtual hospital from a previous exercise, click on **Leave the Floor** and then **Restart the Program** to get to the sign-in window.)
- From the Patient List, select Carrie Richards (Room 303).
- Click on **Go to Nurses' Station**.
- Click on **Chart** and then on **303**.
- Review the **History and Physical**.

1. In the previous exercise, you learned about the following assessment data for failure to thrive. Based on your review of her chart, place an X next to any data that are consistent with failure to thrive in Carrie Richards' case.

_____ a. Weight less than 3rd to 5th percentile

_____ b. Sudden deceleration in growth or weight loss

_____ c. Delay in reaching milestones

_____ d. Decreased muscle mass

_____ e. Muscle hypotonia

_____ f. Wary of caregivers

_____ g. Unresponsive to cuddling

_____ h. Nonnurturing parenting behaviors

_____ i. Avoidance of eye contact or touch

_____ j. Intense watchfulness

_____ k. Sleep disturbance

_____ l. Lack of age-appropriate stranger anxiety

_____ m. Lack of preference for parents

- Click on **Return to Nurses' Station** and then on **303** at the bottom of the screen.
- Click on **Patient Care** and then on **Nurse-Client Interactions**.
- Select and view the video titled **0755: Intervention—Weight**. (*Note:* Check the virtual clock to see whether enough time has elapsed. You can use the fast-forward feature to advance the time by 2-minute intervals if the video is not yet available. Then click again on **Patient Care** and **Nurse-Client Interactions** to refresh the screen.)

2. How should the nurse weigh Carrie Richards? Why is she obtaining the weight before feeding since Carrie has been fussy and seems to want to be fed?

➤ • Now select and view the video titled **0800: Assessment—Fact Finding**. (*Note:* Check the virtual clock to see whether enough time has elapsed. You can use the fast-forward feature to advance the time by 2-minute intervals if the video is not yet available. Then click again on **Patient Care** and **Nurse-Client Interactions** to refresh the screen.)

3. What do you think the nurse is assessing as she observes the mother feeding Carrie Richards?

4. Why is it essential to know that Carrie Richards' mother is able to respond to her infant's cues and correctly interpret them?

5. A nursing care plan has been started for Carrie Richards. One nursing diagnosis is Ineffective coping related to decreased income and lack of support. The goals are for Carrie's mother to identify resources and support systems available to her. What interventions would you anticipate finding in her care plan?

6. What if you noticed that Carrie Richards' mother always had the TV on while feeding Carrie and seemed to pay more attention to the TV than to Carrie? How would you intervene?

7. Envision yourself working with Carrie Richards' mother. How do you feel toward her? What do you think it would be like to carry out this nursing care? (*Hint:* Think about what the term "Rescue Fantasy" means to you.)

Caring for a Young Child with Meningitis

Reading Assignment: The Toddler (Chapter 17, pages 399-413)

The Preschooler (Chapter 18, pages 414-428)

The Child's Experience of Hospitalization (Chapter 21, pages 463-479)

Health Care Adaptations for the Child and Family (Chapter 22, pages 494-495)

The Child with a Sensory or Neurological Condition (Chapter 23, pages 530-531)

Patient: Stephanie Brown, Pediatrics Floor, Room 304

Objectives:

- Describe the pathophysiology of meningitis.
- Discuss risk factors for meningitis.
- List assessment data indicative of meningitis.
- Explain the rationale for treatment of meningitis.
- Develop interventions for caring for a child with meningitis.
- Discuss strategies for supporting a parent and child through diagnosis and treatment.

In this lesson you will learn about the problem of meningitis in a child and the related nursing care. You will focus on a variety of challenges associated with this problem. You may need to review the concepts of growth and development of a young child, as well as teaching-learning principles.

Exercise 1

 Writing Activity

 15 minutes

 1. Explain the pathophysiology of meningitis in terms that a parent would understand. (*Hint:* See page 534 in your textbook for help.)

2. What test is used to diagnose meningitis? What data are consistent with a diagnosis of meningitis?

3. What is nuchal rigidity?

Exercise 2

  CD-ROM Activity

30 minutes

- Sign in to work at Pacific View Regional Hospital on the Pediatrics Floor for Period of Care 1. (*Note:* If you are already in the virtual hospital from a previous exercise, click on **Leave the Floor** and then **Restart the Program** to get to the sign-in window.)
- From the Patient List, select Stephanie Brown (Room 304).
- Click on **Get Report**.
- Click on **Go to Nurses' Station**.
- Click on **Chart** and then on **304**.
- Click on and review the following sections of the chart: **Physician's Notes**, **Emergency Department**, **History and Physical**, and **Nursing Admission**.

1. What assessment data did Stephanie Brown exhibit on admission that would indicate a diagnosis of meningitis?

2. Increased intracranial pressure is a potential concern in a child with meningitis. What changes in vital signs might indicate intracranial pressure and should be reported to the RN?

3. If Stephanie Brown were an infant, what other assessments should you perform?

 - Click on **Return to Nurses' Station** and then on **304**.
- Click on **Take Vital Signs**.
- Review Stephanie Brown's vital signs.

4. Do any of Stephanie Brown's vital signs need to be reported immediately? Why or why not?

- Click on **Chart** and then on **304** to return to Stephanie Brown's chart.
- Click on the **Physician's Orders** tab and review the information given.
- Then click on the **Diagnostic Reports** tab and review the information there.

5. You are to assist the physician with a spinal tap. List your responsibilities.

6. How should you anticipate positioning and supporting Stephanie through the lumbar puncture procedure?

7. Match each of the following physician's orders with its rationale.

Physician's Order	Rationale
_____ Pulse oximetry q4h	a. Baseline (aminoglycosides can cause ototoxicity)
_____ Neuro checks q4h	b. To reduce intracranial pressure
_____ Blood culture for fever above 101 degrees	c. To maintain therapeutic blood level
_____ Audiogram	d. Monitoring of neurologic status
_____ HOB elevated 45 degrees	e. To prevent disease transmission via droplets
_____ Respiratory isolation	f. Assessment for other causative agents
_____ Vancomycin levels	g. Ongoing monitoring of O_2 status

Exercise 3

 CD-ROM Activity

 45 minutes

- Sign in to work at Pacific View Regional Hospital on the Pediatrics Floor for Period of Care 1. (*Note:* If you are already in the virtual hospital from a previous exercise, click on **Leave the Floor** and then **Restart the Program** to get to the sign-in window.)
- From the Patient List, select Stephanie Brown (Room 304).
- Inside Stephanie's room, click on **Go to Nurses' Station** and then on **304**.
- Click on **Patient Care** and complete a focused assessment of Stephanie's neurologic status.
- When you finish your assessment, click on **Leave the Floor**.
- From the Floor Menu, select **Look at Your Preceptor's Evaluations**.
- Next, click on **Examination Report** and review the feedback.

1. Reflect on your assessment skills. Did you miss any areas?

- To return to the Pediatrics Floor, click on **Return to Evaluations** and then on **Return to Menu**.
- From the Floor Menu, click on **Restart the Program**.
- Sign in to work on the Pediatrics Floor for Period of Care 2.
- From the Patient List, select Stephanie Brown.
- Click on **Go to Nurses' Station** and then on **304**.
- Click on **Patient Care** and then on **Nurse-Client Interactions**.
- Select and view the video titled **1120: Preventing Spread of Disease**. (*Note:* Check the virtual clock to see whether enough time has elapsed. You can use the fast-forward feature to advance the time by 2-minute intervals if the video is not yet available. Then click again on **Patient Care** and **Nurse-Client Interactions** to refresh the screen.)

2. CDC guidelines require standard precautions for all types of meningitis, as well as droplet precautions for certain types. What else must be done to effectively implement droplet precautions? (*Hint:* Refer to Appendix A-1 in your textbook: Standard Precautions and Body Substance Isolation Precautions)

3. The above guidelines are implemented immediately and kept in place until 24 hours after antibiotics have been started. Why?

4. Antibiotics are always administered before the culture results come back. Why?

5. What kind of isolation was the nurse in the video using? Was this correct and consistent with the physician's orders?

6. Suppose that you see Stephanie Brown's mother not wearing a mask. When you ask her about this, she says she doesn't need to do anything special because she never leaves Stephanie's room. How would you respond?

7. Every time you walk into the room with your mask on, Stephanie starts to scream. This behavior occurs even when you have observed her through the window quietly playing with her mother before you come in the room. What is going on, and how might you respond?

- Again, click on **Patient Care** and then on **Nurse-Client Interactions**.
- Select and view the video titled **1145: Teaching—Disease Sequelae**. (*Note:* Check the virtual clock to see whether enough time has elapsed. You can use the fast-forward feature to advance the time by 2-minute intervals if the video is not yet available. Then click again on **Patient Care** and **Nurse-Client Interactions** to refresh the screen.)

8. The charge nurse tells you to take care when entering Stephanie Brown's room and when working with her. She also says to keep stimulation to a minimum. What does she mean, and how do you specifically need to behave?

- Click on **Chart** and then on **304**.
- Click on **Physician's Orders**.

9. Is Stephanie Brown on any treatment or medication that may contribute to permanent injury?

10. Review Stephanie Brown's IV orders. Calculate the total volume for 24 hours.

➜ • Click on **Return to Room 304**.
   • Next, click on **Leave the Floor** and then on **Restart the Program**.
   • Sign in to work on the Pediatrics Floor for Period of Care 3.
   • From the Patient List, select Stephanie Brown (Room 304).
   • Click on **Go to Nurses' Station** and then on **304** to go to Stephanie's room.
   • Click on **Patient Care** and then on **Nurse-Client Interactions**.
   • Select and view the video titled **1510: Nurse-Patient Communication**. (*Note:* Check the virtual clock to see whether enough time has elapsed. You can use the fast-forward feature to advance the time by 2-minute intervals if the video is not yet available. Then click again on **Patient Care** and **Nurse-Client Interactions** to refresh the screen.)

11. What is the nurse's assessment and decision in the video?

12. The nurse explains to Stephanie that she is going to apply a local anesthetic. What is a more age-appropriate way of saying this?

13. What is the anesthetic being used? How is it used in order to be most effective? (*Hint:* See page 468 in your textbook.)

14. Note the nurse's interaction with Stephanie Brown and her mother. Why is Stephanie Brown, who is only 3 years old, included in the explanation?

15. At Stephanie Brown's age, how might she perceive her hospital experience? How might she perceive the nurse?

16. How might Stephanie's mother's behavior affect Stephanie's perceptions?

17. From a developmental perspective, what are major fears of children in Stephanie Brown's age group? What behaviors might the child display?

18. What strategies can you use to promote a more positive experience for Stephanie Brown?

19. Let's assume that Stephanie Brown has had a relapse and is now doing worse. Other family members have been taking turns staying with her. She still has an IV and is very restless and irritable. Even the family members are getting irritable, and they express concern about all the babies on the unit that have to be fed and cared for. They worry about Stephanie Brown receiving the care she needs. How will you help them?

LESSON 17

Caring for a Young Child with Cerebral Palsy

Reading Assignment: An Overview of Growth, Development, and Nutrition
(Chapter 15, pages 345-379)
The Toddler (Chapter 17, pages 399-413)
The Preschooler (Chapter 18, pages 414-428)
The Child with a Sensory or Neurological Condition
(Chapter 23, pages 537-540)

Patient: Stephanie Brown, Pediatrics Floor, Room 304

Objectives:

- Describe the behaviors and problems associated with the most common types of cerebral palsy (CP).
- Discuss a range of precipitating factors associated with cerebral palsy.
- Explain the importance of early diagnosis and treatment to the child's optimal level of function.
- Discuss the nursing care needs of a child with cerebral palsy.

Completing this lesson will help you gain an appreciation of the challenges associated with caring for a child who has cerebral palsy—both for parents and for the nurse. You will also explore the issue of encountering cerebral palsy as a condition that coexists with other health problems, the latter being the reason for hospitalization or other health care encounter. You will be working with Stephanie Brown in Room 304.

Exercise 1

 Writing Activity

30 minutes

1. When children are hospitalized for an acute illness, you may find that they also have another disability or chronic illness that could have an effect on the hospitalization or on your care. Think about how you would provide care in such a situation. How do you get information? Who is in charge? Should you involve parents in the same ways you normally do?

2. How do you feel about people with disabilities? Reflect and respond.

3. Consider ideas for teaching parents to promote their child's self-esteem as the child progresses through the stage of initiative versus guilt. What strategies might you suggest?

4. Does your community have a Children with Special Care Needs/Early Intervention Program? What do you think this type of program is about?

5. Visit www.ucp.org and then respond to the following questions:

   a. What did you like or not like about the site?

   b. To whom is this site geared?

   c. What did you learn that was new information?

   d. Would you recommend this site to parents of a child with cerebral palsy? Why or why not?

6. You may have a very general understanding of cerebral palsy. Perhaps you think you have encountered people with this condition in your personal and professional life and remember thinking that they seemed challenging to care for. Describe cerebral palsy.

7. What are some precipitating factors for cerebral palsy?

8. What types of fine and gross motor functions may be affected by cerebral palsy?

9. Early recognition and treatment are important to fostering achievement of optimal development. Why is cerebral palsy often not diagnosed until about 2 years of age?

Exercise 2

 CD-ROM Activity

 30 minutes

- Sign in to work at Pacific View Regional Hospital on the Pediatrics Floor for Period of Care 1. (*Note:* If you are already in the virtual hospital from a previous exercise, click on **Leave the Floor** and then **Restart the Program** to get to the sign-in window.)
- From the Patient List, select Stephanie Brown (Room 304).
- Click on **Get Report** and read the clinical report.
- Click on **Go to Nurses' Station** and then on **304** to go to Stephanie Brown's room.
- Click on **Patient Care** and perform a focused assessment.

1. Based on your assessment of Stephanie Brown, list any behavioral responses she demonstrates that are associated with cerebral palsy.

- Click on **Chart** and then on **304**.
- Click on the **History and Physical** tab.

2. Review Stephanie Brown's history. What might be a precipitating factor in her situation?

3. Think about nursing admissions procedures. What additional information would be especially important to have?

 • Click on **Return to Room 304**.

• Click on **Patient Care** and then on **Nurse-Client Interactions**.

• Select and view the video titled **0750: Caring for the Child with CP**. (*Note:* Check the virtual clock to see whether enough time has elapsed. You can use the fast-forward feature to advance the time by 2-minute intervals if the video is not yet available. Then click again on **Patient Care** and **Nurse-Client Interactions** to refresh the screen.)

4. What should the nurse be doing as she listens to Stephanie Brown's mother explain the problems that Stephanie has associated with cerebral palsy.

5. Should the nurse be supportive of Stephanie Brown's mother implementing the treatments and strategies she uses at home in the hospital? Why or why not?

6. For what problem is Stephanie Brown at risk during her hospitalization? (*Hint:* You will need to consider Stephanie Brown's developmental age.)

 • Click on **Chart** and then on **304**.

• Click on the **Nursing Admission** tab and review for data about Stephanie Brown's development.

7. Hospitalization can still be a time of growth. Explore which developmental tasks Stephanie has achieved and which she has not. Comment on her development.

8. This is a good opportunity to explore Stephanie Brown's development further. One tool is the Denver Developmental Screening Test II (DDST-II). Identify the areas assessed on this test.

9. Parents often express concern about their child's performance when the Denver Developmental Screening Test II is used. Explain the purpose of this test and discuss what a screening test is.

Exercise 3

 CD-ROM Activity

 30 minutes

- Sign in to work at Pacific View Regional Hospital on the Pediatrics Floor for Period of Care 3. (*Note:* If you are already in the virtual hospital from a previous exercise, click on **Leave the Floor** and then **Restart the Program** to get to the sign-in window.)
- From the Patient List, select Stephanie Brown (Room 304).
- Click on **Get Report** and read the clinical report.
- Click on **Go to Nurses' Station**.
- Click on **Chart** and then on **304**.
- Review Stephanie Brown's records, in particular her History and Physical.

1. Match each type of cerebral palsy with its description.

Type	Description
_____ Spastic	a. Rigid flexor and extensor muscles; tremors
_____ Dyskinetic/athetoid	b. Increased deep tendon reflexes, hypertonia, flexion, and scissors gait
_____ Ataxic	c. Slow, writhing uncontrolled and involuntary movements
_____ Mixed	d. Loss of coordination, equilibrium, and kinesthetic sense

2. What type of cerebral palsy does Stephanie Brown have? What are the signs that she manifests?

3. Cerebral palsy can have an impact on many aspects of a child's life. A number of problems can be associated with the behaviors the child manifests. What are some of these problems? (*Note:* Make sure that at least one is a psychosocial concern.)

4. If Stephanie Brown's mother expresses guilt over Stephanie's condition and states that she knows now that she did some things that may have contributed to the condition, how would you respond? (*Hint:* You may want to review your response to question 2 in Exercise 1 of this lesson.)

5. Assume that Stephanie Brown's mother asks you whether you see any signs of mental retardation in her daughter. She is worried that this will develop as Stephanie's disease progresses. What can you tell her? How will you reassure her?

 • Click on **Return to Nurses' Station** and then on **304**.
  • Click on **Patient Care** and then on **Nurse-Client Interactions**.
  • Select and view the video titled **1530: Preventive Measures**. (*Note:* Check the virtual clock to see whether enough time has elapsed. You can use the fast-forward feature to advance the time by 2-minute intervals if the video is not yet available. Then click again on **Patient Care** and **Nurse-Client Interactions** to refresh the screen.)

6. Why does Stephanie Brown require heel cord stretching?

7. What other preventive measures have been integrated into Stephanie Brown's regimen to prevent complications associated with cerebral palsy?

8. What is the nursing role in regard to supporting the mother's implementation of these measures?

9. Explain why nutrition is so important for the child who has cerebral palsy.

10. Nurses are frequently asked for advice. Stephanie Brown's mother sends her daughter to a preschool program but wonders whether it is the best program for her. What advice can you give her?

Caring for a School-Age Child with Diabetes Mellitus

Reading Assignment: The School-Age Child (Chapter 19, pages 429-443)
The Child with a Metabolic Condition (Chapter 30, pages 698-710)

Patient: George Gonzalez, Pediatrics Floor, Room 301

Objectives:

- Review the pathophysiology of diabetes mellitus (DM).
- Compare and contrast type 1 and type 2 diabetes.
- Explain the role of insulin in the metabolism of foods.
- Explain the classic signs of diabetes: polyuria, polydipsia, and polyphagia.
- Discuss management and nursing responsibilities for insulin therapy, diet, exercise, and blood glucose monitoring.
- Contrast hypoglycemia and hyperglycemia with regard to causes, signs and symptoms, and management.
- Explain diabetic ketoacidosis and discuss its management and nursing care.
- Discuss the impact of growth and development on diabetes.

In this lesson you will learn about the problem of meningitis in a child and the related nursing care. You will focus on a variety of challenges associated with this problem. You may need to review the concepts of growth and development of a young child, as well as teaching-learning principles.

Exercise 1

Writing Activity

30 minutes

The assumption is that you have encountered information about diabetes mellitus in your educational experience. Let's begin by going over some key points. (*Hint:* If you run across something with which you are unfamiliar, you may need to take the time to do a little more review.)

1. Describe diabetes mellitus.

2. Differentiate between type 1 and type 2 diabetes mellitus by matching each of the following characteristics to its corresponding type of DM.

Characteristic	**Type of DM**
_____ Most common endocrine disease in children	a. Type 1 diabetes mellitus
_____ Results from destruction of pancreatic beta cells	b. Type 2 diabetes mellitus
_____ Cells unable to use insulin	
_____ Genetic predisposition	
_____ Pancreas unable to produce insulin	
_____ Commonly characterized by obesity	
_____ Prone to ketosis	
_____ Also called noninsulin-dependent diabetes mellitus	
_____ Also called insulin-dependent diabetes mellitus	

3. What symptoms might a child have at the time of diagnosis of diabetes? (*Hint:* Be sure to consider growth and development in your discussion.)

4. What are the signs of the presence of hyperglycemia (diabetes)?

5. How is hyperglycemia treated?

6. Discuss the relationship between exercise and insulin.

7. What is the current thinking about dietary management of diabetes?

8. What are the signs of hypoglycemia?

9. How is hypoglycemia managed?

10. What is HbA1C? Explain its use as a diagnostic and monitoring tool.

11. A combination of a short-acting and an intermediate-acting insulin is often ordered for patients with diabetes. Match each of the following characteristics with its corresponding type of insulin.

Characteristic	Type of Insulin
_____ Onset of 15-30 minutes	a. Regular
_____ Onset of 1-1.5 hours	b. NPH
_____ Peak at 5-10 hours	
_____ Peak at 2-4 hours	
_____ Duration of 6-8 hours	
_____ Duration of 24 hours	

12. Based on the above information, at what time of day would a person who receives NPH insulin in the morning be at greatest risk for a hypoglycemic episode?
   a. Midmorning
   b. Midafternoon
   c. After dinner

Exercise 2

 CD-ROM Activity

 60 minutes

- Sign in to work at Pacific View Regional Hospital on the Pediatrics Floor for Period of Care 1. (*Note:* If you are already in the virtual hospital from another exercise, click on **Leave the Floor** and then **Restart the Program** to get to the sign-in window.)
- From the patient List, select George Gonzalez (Room 301).
- Click on **Go to Nurses' Station**.
- Click on **Chart** and then on **301**.
- Click on the **Emergency Department** tab and review this record.

   1. George Gonzalez has been admitted with a diagnosis of diabetic ketoacidosis (DKA). What does this mean?

2. What signs and symptoms did George Gonzalez manifest on admission to the Emergency Department? Is there a known precipitating factor? What are possible precipitating factors of DKA?

3. What will be the focus of care for the first portion of George Gonzalez's hospitalization for DKA?

4. When treating DKA, what type of insulin is used? Why?

5. Identify any nursing concerns associated with IV administration of insulin.

→ • Continue reviewing the **Emergency Department** record and look for a pattern in George Gonzalez's blood glucose levels.

6. What was George Gonzalez's blood glucose level on admission? What was it after a period of IV therapy with insulin?

➡ • Click on the **History and Physical** tab and review the information given.

7. Why was George Gonzalez at particular risk for development of diabetes mellitus?

8. What ongoing assessments do you need to make when caring for George Gonzalez?

9. Even though blood glucose monitors are used almost exclusively, why is urine testing still performed when diabetic ketoacidosis is the diagnosis?

➡ • Click on **Return to Nurses' Station** and then on **301**.
   • Click on **Patient Care** and complete a head-to-toe assessment.
   • After you have completed the assessment, click on **Leave the Floor**.
   • From the Floor Menu, select **Look at Your Preceptor's Evaluations**.
   • Next, click on **Examination Report** and review the feedback.

10. Note any significant findings and reflect on your performance.

• Click on **Return to Evaluations** and then on **Return to Menu**.

• Click on **Restart the Program** and sign in to work on the Pediatrics Floor for Period of Care 1.

• From the Patient List, select George Gonzalez (Room 301).

• Click **Go to Nurses' Station** and then on **301**.

• Click on **Patient Care** and then on **Nurse-Client Interactions**.

• Select and view the video titled **0730: Supervision—Glucose Testing**. (*Note:* Check the virtual clock to see whether enough time has elapsed. You can use the fast-forward feature to advance the time by 2-minute intervals if the video is not yet available. Then click again on **Patient Care** and **Nurse-Client Interactions** to refresh the screen.)

11. What did the nurse do that facilitated George Gonzalez's honesty about how he tests and how he feels about it?

12. What is the nurse trying to accomplish when she asks George Gonzalez to do his own fingerstick? (*Hint:* Consider the developmental tasks of a school-age child.)

13. How might George Gonzalez's age and interests affect his compliance with treatment?

 • Click **Patient Care** and then **Nurse-Client Interactions**.

• Select and view the video titled **0745: Self-Administering Insulin**. (*Note:* Check the virtual clock to see whether enough time has elapsed. You can use the fast-forward feature to advance the time by 2-minute intervals if the video is not yet available. Then click again on **Patient Care** and **Nurse-Client Interactions** to refresh the screen.)

14. What does the nurse do that is positive as she observes George Gonzalez give himself his injection?

George needs insulin. Before going to the Medication Room, complete any necessary assessments.

 • Click on **MAR** to check the order for insulin; then click on **Return to Room 301**.

• Click on **Medication Room**.

• Using the five rights, prepare the correct dose of insulin for George Gonzalez. When you have prepared the medication, return to George's room and administer it, again following the five rights. (*Hint:* Try to perform these steps on your own. If you need help, refer to pages 26-30 and 37-41 in the **Getting Started** section of this workbook.)

• After administering the insulin, click on **Leave the Floor** and then on **Look at Your Preceptor's Evaluations**.

• Next, click on **Medication Scorecard** and review the feedback.

15. Do you need to do anything differently to satisfactorily complete the procedure? If so, explain.

 • Click on **Return to Evaluations** and then on **Return to Menu**.

• Click on **Restart the Program**.

• Sign in to work on the Pediatrics Floor for Period of Care 1.

• From the Patient List, select George Gonzalez (Room 301).

• Click on **Go to Nurses' Station**.

• Click on **Chart** and then on **301**.

• Click on the **Physician's Orders** tab. Find the order for George Gonzalez's morning dose of insulin.

16. Using this insulin order, describe the steps for drawing up two different insulins into one syringe.

17. Why is short-acting insulin always drawn up first?

18. How should George Gonzalez be advised to rotate injection sites?

Let's jump ahead in virtual time to review and reinforce your insulin administrations skills.

- Click on **Leave the Floor** and then on **Restart the Program**.
- Sign in to work on the Pediatrics Floor for Period of Care 2.
- From the Patient List, select George Gonzalez (Room 301).
- Click on **Go to Nurses' Station**.
- Once again, prepare and administer George Gonzalez's morning dose of insulin. Using the five rights, be sure to check the order, as well as George's current blood glucose level. Perform the proper identification checks before giving the medication.
- After administering the insulin, check your performance by reviewing the preceptor's **Medication Scorecard**.

19. Reflect on your performance. Consider the actual practice you may need in order to feel comfortable with this skill.

20. List the learning needs of patients newly diagnosed with diabetes.

21. Which of the above learning needs do George Gonzalez and his family currently have?

 • To return to the floor, click on **Return to Evaluations**, **Return to Menu**, and **Restart the Program**.
  • Sign in to work on the Pediatrics Floor, again for Period of Care 2.
  • From the Patient List, select George Gonzalez (Room 301).
  • Click on **Go to Nurses' Station** and then on **301**.
  • Click on **Patient Care** and then on **Nurse-Client Interactions**.
  • Select and view the video titled **1115: Teaching—Disease Process**. (*Note:* Check the virtual clock to see whether enough time has elapsed. You can use the fast-forward feature to advance the time by 2-minute intervals if the video is not yet available. Then click again on **Patient Care** and **Nurse-Client Interactions** to refresh the screen.)

22. What are the sequelae of untreated or poorly managed diabetes? Explain why these occur.

Exercise 3

Writing Activity

15 minutes

1. You are a nurse in a physician's office, and you notice that more and more diabetes treatment is taking place on an outpatient basis. Why do you think this is occurring? What are some approaches for responding to learning needs of children such as George Gonzalez?

2. Compare and contrast two or more websites designed for individuals with diabetes and their families. Write about each website's target audience, ease of use, and appropriateness for patients with diabetes and their families. You may do a search and select your own websites or choose from the following established sites:
   - www.diabetes.org
   - www.idcdiabetes.org
   - www.jdrf.org
   - www.niddk.nih.gov

3. Discuss strategies for dealing with the struggles George Gonzalez and his mother seem to be having.

4. Do you think that George Gonzalez is a candidate for an insulin pump? Why or why not? (*Hint:* Consider whether or not you see any ethical issues.)

At this point, you have developed a basic understanding of diabetes in the school-age child. This understanding includes changing needs that occur with growth and development. Proceed to the next lesson to gain more experience helping children learn self-care for diabetes mellitus.

19

Supporting the Child with Diabetes and His Family While Learning Self-Care

Reading Assignment: The School-Age Child (Chapter 19, pages 429-443)
The Child with a Metabolic Condition (Chapter 30, pages 698-710)

Patient: George Gonzalez, Pediatrics Floor, Room 301

Objectives:

- Identify the learning needs of a child newly diagnosed with diabetes mellitus.
- Develop a developmentally appropriate plan for teaching a child independence with care of diabetes.
- Explore the need for information, readiness, capability, and motivation as significant factors in the teaching-learning process.
- Differentiate roles of the child and the parent in managing the child's diabetes.

In this lesson you will focus on the teaching aspect in the care of the child with diabetes. You will consider learning needs according to developmental stage and parental responsibilities, along with the dynamic nature of supervision and self-care. You may need to review developmental issues associated with various age groups. You may also need to review the teaching-learning process since you will be applying these principles throughout your work.

Exercise 1

Writing Activity

45 minutes

1. Review information about learning needs in your textbook. How will you determine the learning needs of a child with diabetes and his family? What are your general thoughts about the influence of different developmental stages? (*Hint:* You do not need to break it down into age groups.)

2. What are the roles and responsibilities of the family in care?

 3. What are some care issues if the child with diabetes is a toddler? What might you suggest to parents? (*Hint:* Refer to Chapter 16 in your textbook.)

 4. What are some care issues if the child with diabetes is a preschooler? What might you suggest to parents in this case? (*Hint:* Refer to Chapter 17 in your textbook.)

5. What are some care issues if the child with diabetes is of school-age. What might you suggest to parents? (*Hint:* Refer to Chapter 19 in your textbook.)

 6. What are some care issues if the child with diabetes is an adolescent? What might you suggest to parents? (*Hint:* Refer to Chapter 20 in your textbook.)

7. You are working with a family whose child was recently diagnosed with diabetes. List several areas that you would want to discuss about diabetes in general.

8. Describe the "honeymoon" phase of diabetes. Why is this significant to parent teaching?

9. What would you do to explain the relationships among food, exercise, and insulin in a way that would be meaningful to parents?

10. Health maintenance and regular visits with health care providers are important, even when the child is doing well. Discuss the issue of who (parent, child, or both) should be in attendance at an office visit.

11. What barriers are there in providing optimal outpatient care for the child with diabetes and the family?

12. You are assisting a nurse who is working with the mother of a child newly diagnosed with diabetes. You observe the teary-eyed parent with an orange and a syringe. How would you respond?

13. Discuss the advantages of diabetes groups or camps for children.

Exercise 2

 CD-ROM Activity

 30 minutes

- Sign in to work at Pacific View Regional Hospital on the Pediatrics Floor for Period of Care 1. (*Note:* If you are already in the virtual hospital from a previous exercise, click on **Leave the Floor** and then **Restart the Program** to get to the sign-in window.)
- From the Patient List, select George Gonzalez (Room 301).
- Click on **Go to Nurses' Station** and then on **301**.
- Click on **Patient Care** and then on **Nurse-Client Interactions**.
- Select and view the video titled **0730: Supervision—Glucose Testing**. (*Note:* Check the virtual clock to see whether enough time has elapsed. You can use the fast-forward feature to advance the time by 2-minute intervals if the video is not yet available. Then click again on **Patient Care** and **Nurse-Client Interactions** to refresh the screen.)

1. Is George Gonzalez physically capable of being responsible for his own blood glucose testing? Comment on his skill and knowledge level for glucose testing.

2. What are some possible reasons that George Gonzalez may be noncompliant with blood glucose testing?

3. What does the nurse do that is effective? What other interventions can be offered?

4. Identify information that is necessary for families to understand about insulin.

5. Identify effective techniques to use for teaching insulin administration to parents and children. Provide rationales where appropriate.

6. What are possible barriers to learning injection techniques?

7. List several issues associated with site selection and rotation that should be discussed with George Gonzalez and his family.

8. How should site selection be considered in relation to absorption?

9. Be creative. Develop a strategy for keeping track of site rotations.

 • Click on **Patient Care** and then on **Nurse-Client Interactions**.

• Select and view the video titled **0745: Self-Administering Insulin**. (*Note:* Check the virtual clock to see whether enough time has elapsed. You can use the fast-forward feature to advance the time by 2-minute intervals if the video is not yet available. Then click again on **Patient Care** and **Nurse-Client Interactions** to refresh the screen.)

10. Evaluate George Gonzalez's performance and comment on anything else you need to do with him to improve his performance.

Exercise 3

 CD-ROM Activity

 30 minutes

- Sign in to work at Pacific View Regional Hospital on the Pediatrics Floor for Period of Care 2. (*Note:* If you are already in the virtual hospital from a previous exercise, click on **Leave the Floor** and then **Restart the Program** to get to the sign-in window.)
- From the Patient List, select George Gonzalez (Room 301).
- Click on **Go to Nurses' Station** and then on **301**.
- Click on **Patient Care** and then on **Nurse-Client Interactions**.
- Select and view the video titled **1115: Teaching—Disease Process**. (*Note:* Check the virtual clock to see whether enough time has elapsed. You can use the fast-forward feature to advance the time by 2-minute intervals if the video is not yet available. Then click again on **Patient Care** and **Nurse-Client Interactions** to refresh the screen.)

1. Evaluate George Gonzalez's understanding of his condition and management of hypoglycemia.

2. What is his mother's level of understanding?

3. Given the responses of George Gonzalez and his mother, is there a need for teaching in this area? If so, what type of teaching needs to be done?

• Click again on **Patient Care** and then on **Nurse-Client Interactions**.

- Select and view the video titled **1130: Teaching—Managing Symptoms**. (*Note:* Check the virtual clock to see whether enough time has elapsed. You can use the fast-forward feature to advance the time by 2-minute intervals if the video is not yet available. Then click again on **Patient Care** and **Nurse-Client Interactions** to refresh the screen.)

4. Do you think George and his mother understand the concept of managing symptoms? Explain your answer.

5. What should the nurse do based on this assessment of George and his mother's level of understanding?

6. Nothing has been said about record keeping. What would you suggest?

Let's jump ahead in virtual time to observe a nurse-patient interaction that occurs later in the day.

 • Click on **Leave the Floor** and then on **Restart the Program**.

- Sign in to work at Pacific View Regional Hospital on the Pediatrics Floor for Period of Care 3.
- From the Patient List, select George Gonzalez (Room 301).
- Click on **Go to Nurses' Station** and then on **301**.
- Click on **Patient Care** and then on **Nurse-Client Interactions**.
- Select and view the video titled **1500: Teaching—Diabetic Diet**. (*Note:* Check the virtual clock to see whether enough time has elapsed. You can use the fast-forward feature to advance the time by 2-minute intervals if the video is not yet available. Then click again on **Patient Care** and **Nurse-Client Interactions** to refresh the screen.)

7. What is George Gonzalez's diet order? What are the recommendations of the dietitian?

8. Evaluate the nurse's teaching with regard to diet. What did she do well? What could she have explained better?

9. Is there anything that the nurse should pursue with George Gonzalez's mother?

→ • Click on **Patient Care** and then on **Nurse-Client Interactions**.
  • Select and view the video titled **1535: Teaching—Effects of Exercise**. (*Note:* Check the virtual clock to see whether enough time has elapsed. You can use the fast-forward feature to advance the time by 2-minute intervals if the video is not yet available. Then click again on **Patient Care** and **Nurse-Client Interactions** to refresh the screen.)

10. Discuss the effects of physical activity on blood sugar levels. Consider times of day when George Gonzalez might have more activity than others.

11. What should George Gonzalez be advised to do in relation to activity?

12. Based on the potential complications discussed in question 10, do you think it would be better if George Gonzalez did not exercise? Explain your response. (*Hint:* Be sure to consider growth and development as a factor.)

20

Caring for a Teen with an Eating Disorder

Reading Assignment: The Adolescent (Chapter 20, pages 444-462)
The Child with an Emotional or Behavioral Condition
(Chapter 32, pages 739-741)

Patient: Tiffany Sheldon, Pediatrics Floor, Room 305

Objectives:

- Compare and contrast description, etiology, and typical behaviors associated with anorexia nervosa and bulimia nervosa.
- Discuss the physiologic impacts of anorexia nervosa and bulimia nervosa.
- Discuss the multidisciplinary approach necessary for treatment of eating disorders.
- Explore the challenges of providing nursing care for patients with anorexia nervosa or bulimia nervosa.

In this lesson you will explore a variety of challenges associated with caring for a teen with an eating disorder. You will care for Tiffany Sheldon, a 14-year-old with a history of eight admissions in the past 2 years for complications associated with anorexia nervosa. You will learn that helping a patient manage an eating disorder requires intensive multidisciplinary effort.

Exercise 1

 Writing Activity

🕐 30 minutes

1. Match each characteristic listed below with its corresponding eating disorder—anorexia nervosa, bulimia nervosa, or both. (*Hint:* Although some characteristics may seem to overlap, most are usually associated more closely with one problem rather than the other. In those cases, choose the problem most closely associated with the characteristic.)

Characteristic	Type of Eating Disorder
_____ Deliberate refusal of food to maintain body weight	a. Anorexia nervosa
_____ Recurrent episodes of binging and a sense of loss of control	b. Bulimia nervosa
_____ Misuse of laxatives and/or diuretics	c. Both anorexia and bulimia
_____ Amenorrhea	
_____ Overconcern with body image, though not distorted	
_____ Body image that is contrary to reality	
_____ Ritualistic eating pattern	
_____ Binge eating and purging	
_____ Muscle wasting, dull and brittle hair, presence of lanugo	
_____ Electrolyte imbalance	
_____ Tooth erosion	
_____ Self-induced vomiting	
_____ Risk factor: participation in sports, dance, or gymnastics	
_____ Cardiac arrhythmias	
_____ Excessive exercise	
_____ Excessive influence of body weight on self-evaluation	
_____ History of family dysfunction	
_____ Weight of less than 85% of what is expected	

2. Give an example of an eating pattern that might be found in a person with anorexia nervosa. What often underlies such behavior?

3. How is it believed that family function and culture play into the problem of eating disorders?

4. What are some secondary gains achieved through eating disorders? (*Hint:* Secondary gains are perceived benefits other than weight loss that the patient gets from his or her disease.)

5. Nurses in schools or other community settings may play several roles with teens who have anorexia nervosa. Discuss one of the primary roles.

6. Assume that you are working in a community setting and a teen says to you, "I have to tell you something, but you can't tell anyone." How would you respond? What would your responsibilities be?

Exercise 2

 CD-ROM Activity

 30 minutes

- Sign in to work at Pacific View Regional Hospital on the Pediatrics Floor for Period of Care 1. (*Note:* If you are already in the virtual hospital from a previous exercise, click on **Leave the Floor** and then **Restart the Program** to get to the sign-in window.)
- From the Patient List, select Tiffany Sheldon (Room 305).
- Click on **Go to Nurses' Station**.
- Click on **Chart** and then on **305**.
- Click on and review the **Nursing Admission** and the **History and Physical**.

1. What in Tiffany Sheldon's history is indicative of her diagnosis of anorexia nervosa?

2. Did you identify family crisis (divorce of parents) as a precipitating factor in Tiffany Sheldon's situation? Did you include the fact that she is an "A" student in your list? Why should you see these factors as red flags?

 • Click on **Return to Nurses' Station** and then on **305** at the bottom of the screen.
   • Click on **Patient Care** and complete a head-to-toe assessment, noting data that are consistent with anorexia nervosa.

3. Based on your assessment, which factors stand out for you? The patient's physical appearance? The systemic problems? How much does nutritional status affect the total patient?

 • Click on **Patient Care** and then on **Nurse-Client Interactions**.
   • Select and view the video titled **0730: Initial Assessment**. (*Note:* Check the virtual clock to see whether enough time has elapsed. You can use the fast-forward feature to advance the time by 2-minute intervals if the video is not yet available. Then click again on **Patient Care** and **Nurse-Client Interactions** to refresh the screen.)

4. Tiffany Sheldon has been described as having a flat affect, being withdrawn, and avoiding eye contact. How would you describe her behavior at the time of this video interaction?

5. What is the most effective form of communication to use with Tiffany Sheldon?

6. Is there anything in the video that you need to report? If so, what?

7. In addition to the nursing assessment, what multidimensional assessments and interventions are needed in order to develop an appropriate plan of care for Tiffany Sheldon?

 • Again, click on **Patient Care** and then on **Nurse-Client Interactions**.
• Select and view the video titled **0800: Coordinating Care**. (*Note:* Check the virtual clock to see whether enough time has elapsed. You can use the fast-forward feature to advance the time by 2-minute intervals if the video is not yet available. Then click again on **Patient Care** and **Nurse-Client Interactions** to refresh the screen.)

8. How do you think Tiffany Sheldon might respond to being told that she will be seen by an Eating Disorders Team?

9. What is the nurse's role in identifying and/or coordinating care and services that Tiffany Sheldon requires during her inpatient stay?

Exercise 3

 CD-ROM Activity

 45 minutes

The first order of business with a patient who has anorexia nervosa is to correct any fluid and electrolyte imbalances. Keep this in mind as you work through this exercise.

- Sign in to work at Pacific View Regional Hospital on the Pediatrics Floor for Period of Care 1. (*Note:* If you are already in the virtual hospital from a previous exercise, click on **Leave the Floor** and then **Restart the Program** to get to the sign-in window.)
- From the Patient List, select Tiffany Sheldon (Room 305).
- Click on **Go to Nurses' Station**.
- Click on **Chart** and then on **305**.
- Click on and review the **Physician's Orders** and the **Laboratory Reports**.

1. What do Tiffany Sheldon's lab results tell you about her fluid and electrolyte status? Report on the ones that give you specific information.

2. What is being done to assess for and manage Tiffany Sheldon's fluid and electrolyte imbalance?

3. Tiffany Sheldon did not have a pH level done. A patient with anorexia nervosa is at risk for metabolic acidosis. What would happen to the pH in this instance?

4. List the objective assessment data that indicate Tiffany Sheldon is dehydrated.

5. Why is Tiffany Sheldon on a cardiac monitor?

6. Tiffany Sheldon is receiving IV fluid with potassium chloride added. What is the order? What are the nursing responsibilities before and during potassium administration?

7. You need to be familiar with care plans for common problems associated with anorexia nervosa. Work on the following problem.

   a. Identify a generic nursing diagnosis for hydration problems in patients with anorexia nervosa.

   b. Now rewrite your nursing diagnosis so that it accurately reflects Tiffany Sheldon's situation.

Next, begin thinking about how adequate caloric intake is achieved.

- Click on **Return to Nurse's Station** and then on **Leave the Floor**.
- From the Floor Menu, select **Restart the Program**.
- Sign in to work at Pacific View Regional Hospital on the Pediatrics Floor for Period of Care 2.
- From the Patient List, select Tiffany Sheldon (Room 305).
- Click on **Go to Nurses' Station** and then on **305** at the bottom of the screen.
- Click on **Patient Care** and then on **Nurse-Client Interactions**.
- Select and view the video titled **1115: Managing Anorexia Nervosa**. (*Note:* Check the virtual clock to see whether enough time has elapsed. You can use the fast-forward feature to advance the time by 2-minute intervals if the video is not yet available. Then click again on **Patient Care** and **Nurse-Client Interactions** to refresh the screen.)

8. Discuss the cultural beliefs and personal perceptions that influence the development of eating disorders. Consider both males and females in your discussion.

9. What is the value of an eating contract for Tiffany Sheldon?

10. What is the rationale for including diet orders as part of the eating contract?

11. Calculate Tiffany Sheldon's daily caloric needs.

* Once again, click on **Patient Care** and then on **Nurse-Client Interactions**.
* Select and view the video titled **1130: Monitoring Compliance**. (*Note:* Check the virtual clock to see whether enough time has elapsed. You can use the fast-forward feature to advance the time by 2-minute intervals if the video is not yet available. Then click again on **Patient Care** and **Nurse-Client Interactions** to refresh the screen.)

12. Why have the measures cited in the video been put into Tiffany's eating contract?

13. What supportive interventions might the nurse provide to help Tiffany Sheldon remain compliant?

Now, consider the emotional aspects of Tiffany Sheldon's care.

* Click on **Leave the Floor** and then **Restart the Program**.
* Sign in to work at Pacific View Regional Hospital on the Pediatrics Floor for Period of Care 3.
* From the Patient List, select Tiffany Sheldon (Room 305).
* Click on **Go to Nurses' Station** and then on **305** at the bottom of the screen.
* Click on **Patient Care** and then on **Nurse-Client Interactions**.
* Select and view the video titled **1500: Relapse—Contributing Factors**. (*Note:* Check the virtual clock to see whether enough time has elapsed. You can use the fast-forward feature to advance the time by 2-minute intervals if the video is not yet available. Then click again on **Patient Care** and **Nurse-Client Interactions** to refresh the screen.)

14. What does Tiffany Sheldon say in regard to what has caused her relapse? What recent events, if any, may have contributed to her having an acute episode of her anorexia nervosa?

15. What did the psychiatrist do to effectively elicit Tiffany Sheldon's concerns?

→ • Click on **Patient Care** and then on **Nurse-Client Interactions**.
  • Select and view the video titled **1530: Facilitating Success**. (*Note:* Check the virtual clock to see whether enough time has elapsed. You can use the fast-forward feature to advance the time by 2-minute intervals if the video is not yet available. Then click again on **Patient Care** and **Nurse-Client Interactions** to refresh the screen.)

16. What does Tiffany Sheldon say about her progress?

17. What multidimensional factors will contribute to Tiffany Sheldon's ability to comply with the eating contract that has been developed? What barriers may be present?

18. A patient with an eating disorder may not like the sensations associated with refeeding. Develop several strategies to help Tiffany Sheldon overcome barriers to the success of her treatment plan.

19. Let's assume that Tiffany Sheldon refuses to eat and her condition puts her at even greater health risk. The hospital is awaiting a court order for a feeding tube. Tiffany will need to be restrained if the order is implemented. How would you handle this situation? What would be your responsibilities as a nurse? (*Hint:* You may want to refer to a fundamentals of nursing textbook.)

Note: Generally, when the facilities are available, patients with eating disorders are transferred to the Eating Disorders Unit, where professionals are highly skilled and experienced with this area of care. However, this may not be the case in all settings; thus all nurses need to be aware of the problems, the risks, and the usual approaches to treatment of eating disorders. You will have accomplished this by completing this lesson.

LESSON 21

Emergency Care for a Child with Head Trauma

Reading Assignment: The Child's Experience of Hospitalization (Chapter 21, pages 463-480)

The Child with a Sensory or Neurological Condition (Chapter 23, pages 542-545)

Patient: Tommy Douglas, Pediatrics Floor, Room 302

Objectives:

- Consider factors that may create a stressful environment in emergency care.
- Discuss nursing interventions supportive to the child and family who are experiencing emergency care.
- Discuss the concept of "across the room" assessment and priority setting for a child in the emergency department.
- Explore the implications of growth and development in emergency care.
- Explore medications frequently used in traumatic emergency situations.
- Identify priority concerns related to head injury.

In this lesson you will explore the role of the nurse in caring for a child in an emergency situation. More often than not, the priority needs of the child will be physiologic, but the psychosocial care for family cannot be ignored. Parents have many support needs that sometimes are pushed aside during the acute phase of the visit. You will learn general strategies for dealing with such issues. You will be working with 6-year-old Tommy Douglas, who has arrived in the emergency department after a blunt trauma injury.

Exercise 1

 Writing Activity

 30 minutes

1. List and explain several factors that can contribute to a stressful environment for a child who is brought to the emergency department after a traumatic event.

2. For each of the factors you listed above, develop a nursing intervention to minimize stress. If you have had experience in such an environment (even during an observation), you have an opportunity to be creative here.

3. What do you think is meant by the notion of "assessment from across the room"? Identify some assessments that can be made in this manner.

4. Rank the following care items in order of priority by numbering from 1 (highest priority) to 7 (lowest priority).

Care Item	Priority Ranking
Trauma scoring	
Assessment of child's coping	
Circulatory assessment	
History of injury	
Breathing assessment	
Airway assessment	
Signs of other injury	

5. Considering your personal knowledge of growth and development, select one age group that you think would be challenging to care for. Explain your reason and use a specific example in your response.

6. Which of the following are the top two concerns of children when confronted with emergency care?

   _____ a. Fear of body intrusion

   _____ b. Fear of the unknown

   _____ c. Pain

   _____ d. Separation

   _____ e. Unfamiliar environment

7. Parents and caregivers need a great deal of support. Nurses need to be able to anticipate fears and anxieties in order to craft careful communication to elicit and respond to concerns. What are some common fears or concerns parents have when their child is brought to the emergency department?

8. Parents may feel pushed aside in the emergency department. How can the nurse deal with this problem? Consider what can be done while care is given and what other measures another staff member could provide.

Exercise 2

 CD-ROM Activity

 45 minutes

You are an LPN who has been hired to work in the Pediatrics Unit. Because so many children come to the unit via the Emergency Department, your unit manager has assigned you to spend the day in the ED to learn about a child and his family's experiences there.

- Sign in to work at Pacific View Regional Hospital on the Pediatrics Floor for Period of Care 1. (*Note:* If you are already in the virtual hospital from a previous exercise, click on **Leave the Floor** and then **Restart the Program** to get to the sign-in window.)
- From the Patient List, select Tommy Douglas (Room 302).
- Click on **Go to Nurses' Station**.
- Click on **Chart** and then on **302**.
- Click on and review the **Emergency Department** and **Physician's Orders** sections.

1. Review the circumstances behind Tommy Douglas' admission. Include such information as the nature of his injury and the people involved.

2. What are the priorities for care for Tommy Douglas?

3. Define ventriculostomy. What is the purpose of this procedure? (*Hint:* Try to identify key parts of the word that can help you with the definition. If necessary, you may refer to a medical dictionary).

4. A priority concern for Tommy Douglas is increased intracranial pressure. List the assessment areas that would indicate increasing intracranial pressure.

5. What changes in vital signs are indicative of increasing intracranial pressure?

→ • Return to the **Emergency Department** record in the chart. Check Tommy's admission vital signs.

6. Compare Tommy Douglas' vital signs to those of a healthy 6-year-old. How do they compare?

7. Do his vital signs reflect increased intracranial pressure?

8. The nurse you are shadowing tells you that abnormal posturing is a sign of brain damage. Explain the differences between decerebrate and decorticate posturing.

➡ • Click on and review the **History and Physical** tab for evidence of abnormal posturing.

9. Does Tommy Douglas manifest abnormal posturing at this point? (*Hint:* Changes may continue to develop as edema and bleeding in the brain increase.)

10. Why is Tommy Douglas receiving bolus infusions?

➡ • Click the **Physician's Orders** tab and review the information given.

11. Review Tommy Douglas' initial medication orders (from admission on Tuesday through Wednesday morning). List the medications ordered and give a rationale for each order.

➡ • Click on **Return to Nurses' Station**.
   • Click on the **Drug** icon in the lower left corner of the screen.
   • Review the medications ordered for Tommy Douglas.

12. You should note that $NaHCO_3$ is incompatible with both dopamine and norepinephrine. What does this mean in regard to administration?

13. Medications are often ordered STAT and have to be given quickly. How much time is generally available in which to give a drug ordered this way? (*Hint:* You may need to refer to a fundamentals of nursing textbook.)

You won't be administering critical care medications during your time in the Emergency Department. However, you do have the opportunity to practice medication administration in the virtual setting of Pacific View Regional Hospital. Select one of the medications that need to be administered during this period of care and complete the following steps to prepare and administer it.

- Click on **Return to Nurses' Station** and then on **Medication Room**.
- Using the five rights, select, prepare, and administer the medication to be given. When you have finished the preparation, return to Tommy Douglas' room and administer the medication. (*Hint:* Although you should be getting more comfortable with the steps of preparing and administering medications, remember that you can refer to pages 26-30 and 37-41 in the **Getting Started** section if you need help.)
- To obtain feedback, click on **Leave the Floor**.
- Click on **Look at Your Preceptor's Evaluations** and then on **Medication Scorecard**.

14. Review the feedback on your Medication Scorecard. Are there any areas in which you need to make changes? If so, select another medication ordered for Tommy Douglas and practice the procedure again.

15. Reflect on your experience and comment on nursing responsibilities for medication administration in the Emergency Department.

• To return to the Pediatrics Floor, click on **Return to Evaluations**, **Return to Menu**, and **Restart the Program**.
• Sign in to work on the Pediatrics Floor for Period of Care 1.
• From the Patient List, select Tommy Douglas (Room 302).
• Click on **Go to Nurses' Station**.
• Click on **Chart** and then on **302**.
• Click on and review the **Physician's Orders** and **Nursing Admission**.

16. The physician has ordered a rate increase for norepinephrine. At what rate was the drug running? To what rate has it been increased?

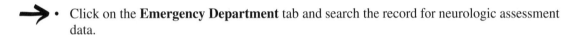 • Click on the **Emergency Department** tab and search the record for neurologic assessment data.

17. Describe the Glasgow Coma Scale (GCS).

18. What significant neurologic data did you find in Tommy Douglas' Emergency Department record?

19. Tommy Douglas is being stabilized in preparation for transfer to the Intensive Care Unit, and a cerebral perfusion scan is performed. What is the purpose of this test?

Exercise 3

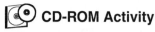 **CD-ROM Activity**

 30 minutes

1. It is determined that Tommy Douglas will not be going to the Intensive Care Unit as planned. He is instead being transferred to the Pediatric Unit for end-of-life care. Explain why you think this decision was made.

 • Sign in to work at Pacific View Regional Hospital on the Pediatrics Floor for Period of Care 1. (*Note:* If you are already in the virtual hospital from a previous exercise, click on **Leave the Floor** and then **Restart the Program** to get to the sign-in window.)

• From the Patient List, select Tommy Douglas (Room 302).

• Click on **Go to Nurses' Station** and then on **302** at the bottom of the screen.

• Click on **Patient Care** and complete a focused neurologic assessment of Tommy Douglas. Chart your findings in the EPR. (*Hint:* If you need help entering data in the EPR, refer to pages 15-16 in the **Getting Started** section of this workbook.)

• To obtain feedback, click **Leave the Floor** and then **Look at Your Preceptor's Evaluations**.

• Select **Examination Report** and review your evaluation.

2. Reflect on the completeness of your focused assessment of Tommy's neurologic status.

• To return to the Pediatrics Floor, click on **Return to Evaluations**, **Return to Menu**, and **Restart the Program**.

- Sign in to work on the Pediatrics Floor for Period of Care 1.
- From the Patient List, select Tommy Douglas (Room 302).
- Click on **Go to Nurses' Station** and then on **302** at the bottom of the screen.
- Click on **Patient Care** and then **Nurse-Client Interactions**.
- Select and view the video titled **0730: Assessment—Neurological**. (*Note:* Check the virtual clock to see whether enough time has elapsed. You can use the fast-forward feature to advance the time by 2-minute intervals if the video is not yet available. Then click again on **Patient Care** and **Nurse-Client Interactions** to refresh the screen.)

3. What was Tommy's GCS score?

4. Consider how well the nurse explained the use and meaning of the GCS to Tommy's parents. Do you think the parents found support during this interaction? What, if anything, would you have done differently?

 • Click again on **Patient Care** and then on **Nurse-Client Interactions**.

- Select and view the video titled **0745: Intervention—Airway**. (*Note:* Check the virtual clock to see whether enough time has elapsed. You can use the fast-forward feature to advance the time by 2-minute intervals if the video is not yet available. Then click again on **Patient Care** and **Nurse-Client Interactions** to refresh the screen.)

5. Tommy Douglas is on a ventilator. What is a ventilator used for? How would you expect Tommy's ventilator to be set?

6. How would you explain to Tommy's parents what the ventilator is doing?

- Once again, click on **Patient Care** and then on **Nurse-Client Interactions**.
- Select and view the video titled **0800: Intervention—Stabilizing Blood Pressure**. (*Note:* Check the virtual clock to see whether enough time has elapsed. You can use the fast-forward feature to advance the time by 2-minute intervals if the video is not yet available. Then click again on **Patient Care** and **Nurse-Client Interactions** to refresh the screen.)

7. Tommy's blood pressure is low. Explain why fluids help to maintain blood pressure.

Tommy Douglas will be receiving end-of-life care. Continue to the next lesson to learn about nursing care for the parents and family of a child who is dying.

LESSON **22**

Providing Support for Families Experiencing the Loss of a Child

Reading Assignment: The Child with a Sensory or Neurological Condition
(Chapter 23, pages 542-545)
The Child with a Condition of the Blood, Blood-Forming
Organs, or Lymphatic System (Chapter 26, pages 627-631)

Patient: Tommy Douglas, Pediatrics Floor, Room 302

Objectives:

- Explore the range of reactions that may occur when parents are told there is no hope of saving their child's life.
- Discuss the role of hospital ethics committees.
- Discuss nursing responsibilities associated with organ donation.
- Discuss the concept of "allowing" a child to die.
- Identify strategies to support parents and other children as a child dies.

In this lesson you will explore circumstances that may occur in hospital settings around a traumatic event resulting in certainty of death. Care for parents and other family members is the major focus during this time of hospice care. You will continue to work with the family of 6-year-old Tommy Douglas as he dies.

Exercise 1

Writing Activity

30 minutes

"Allowing" a child to die is a very difficult concept. Parents go through several stages of emotion as their child dies.

1. Discuss what parents go through when their child experiences a life-threatening injury or illness that then becomes terminal.

2. Parents frequently need to talk about what is happening while their child is dying. Why?

3. What occurs in the dying process that are indications of imminent death?

22 ————————————————

4. Assume that you enter the room and find parents sobbing as they sit with their dying child. Does this mean you have not been effective with your teaching and care? What can you do for these parents?

5. How might you guide parents at the time of death? (*Hint:* Remember that allowing a child to die is tremendously difficult for parents and is often perceived as out of the order of natural events.)

6. What are your thoughts about how you would provide care for the family members after the death of the child?

7. How do you think you might react to caring for a dying child and the family? Do you think you could be effective? Explain your response.

8. Review the nursing care plan for parents found on pages 629-630 of your textbook. Reflect on the nursing interventions listed. Can you see yourself, at this point, carrying out each intervention? Which ones would you find difficult? What can you do to prepare yourself for providing this sort of nursing care?

9. Discuss ways that nurses who care for dying children cope with their own grief.

Exercise 2

 CD-ROM Activity

 45 minutes

- Sign in to work at Pacific View Regional Hospital on the Pediatrics Floor for Period of Care 2. (*Note:* If you are already in the virtual hospital from a previous exercise, click on **Leave the Floor** and then **Restart the Program** to get to the sign-in window.)
- From the Patient List, select Tommy Douglas (Room 302).
- Click on **Go to Nurses' Station** and then on **302** at the bottom of the screen.
- Click on **Patient Care** and then on **Nurse-Client Interactions**.
- Select and view the video titled **1115: The Family (Care) Conference**. (*Note:* Check the virtual clock to see whether enough time has elapsed. You can use the fast-forward feature to advance the time by 2-minute intervals if the video is not yet available. Then click again on **Patient Care** and **Nurse-Client Interactions** to refresh the screen.)

1. Tommy Douglas has been certified as "brain dead," and a family conference has been held to inform his parents that he will not be helped by further intervention. Who are the usual participants in such a conference? What does each person bring to the discussion?

2. What intervention can the nurse provide to the parents after the family conference?

3. What if Tommy's parents say that they want him to live "at all costs"? How would you feel about this?

4. Discuss how your response to the previous question might affect your care for Tommy's parents.

→ • Again, click on **Patient Care** and then on **Nurse-Client Interactions**.

• Select and view the video titled **1130: Decision—Organ Donation**. (*Note:* Check the virtual clock to see whether enough time has elapsed. You can use the fast-forward feature to advance the time by 2-minute intervals if the video is not yet available. Then click again on **Patient Care** and **Nurse-Client Interactions** to refresh the screen.)

5. Tommy's parents have agreed to organ donation. Does this provide evidence of progression with anticipatory grieving?

6. Visit the website for United Network for Organ Sharing (www.unos.org) and discuss the criteria for donation and management of a potential donor.

- Click on **Chart** and then on **302**.
- Click on the **Physician's Orders** tab and review.

7. Discuss the kind of care that is being provided for Tommy Douglas during this time.

8. Tommy Douglas is to receive hospice care. Compare palliative and hospice care. (*Hint:* You may want to refer to your medical dictionary.)

Let's check in on Tommy Douglas' family a little later in the day.

- Click on **Leave the Floor** and then on **Restart the Program**.
- Sign in to work on the Pediatrics Floor for Period of Care 3.
- From the Patient List, select Tommy Douglas (Room 302).
- Click on **Go to Nurses' Station** and then on **302** at the bottom of the screen.
- Click on **Patient Care** and then on **Nurse-Client Interactions**.
- Select and view the video titled **1500: Nurse—Family Communication**. (*Note:* Check the virtual clock to see whether enough time has elapsed. You can use the fast-forward feature to advance the time by 2-minute intervals if the video is not yet available. Then click again on **Patient Care** and **Nurse-Client Interactions** to refresh the screen.)

9. Evaluate the nurse's approach to dealing with a family in crisis. Did the nurse demonstrate empathy? If so, how?

10. Is the nurse's body language congruent with his verbal communication?

11. Present an alternative to the nurse's approach if you believe it is indicated.

You need to learn more about Tommy's family, most importantly whether or not he has siblings.

→ • Click on **Nurses' Station**.
   • Click on **Chart** and then on **302**.
   • Click on **History and Physical** and review Tommy's family configuration.

12. Did you find information about siblings? If yes, what do you know? Do you need more information?

→ • Click on the **Nursing Admission** tab and review the information given.

13. What else did you learn about siblings?

• Click on **Return to Nurses' Station** and then on **302** at the bottom of the screen.
- Click on **Patient Care** and then on **Nurse-Client Interactions**.
- Select and view the video titled **1515: The Grieving Family**. (*Note:* Check the virtual clock to see whether enough time has elapsed. You can use the fast-forward feature to advance the time by 2-minute intervals if the video is not yet available. Then click again on **Patient Care** and **Nurse-Client Interactions** to refresh the screen.)

14. How are siblings of a dying child likely to view death?

15. For parents who have lost a child, what anticipatory guidance could you offer for dealing with other children in their family?

This lesson has given you the opportunity to consider care of the terminally ill child and many of the issues that might arise. This experience will help you to be more effective with your nursing care in similar situations—and it will help you take better care of yourself.